An Assessment of State Voting Processes

Preparing for Elections During a Pandemic

JENNIFER KAVANAGH, QUENTIN E. HODGSON, C. BEN GIBSON,
SAMANTHA CHERNEY

RAND CORPORATION

For more information on this publication, visit www.rand.org/t/RRA112-8

Library of Congress Cataloging-in-Publication Data is available for this publication.
ISBN: 978-1-9774-0554-8

Published by the RAND Corporation, Santa Monica, Calif.

Cover image: Bill Oxford/Getty Images

Preface

In this report, we summarize state election laws on voter registration, remote voting, and early voting, and we discuss the potential implications of these laws for the execution of the November 2020 general election under conditions brought on by the coronavirus disease 2019 (COVID-19) pandemic.[1] We consider how easily states will be able to hold elections while incorporating social distancing and remote processes that reduce person-to-person contact. This report is intended to inform state legislatures and election officials as they prepare for the 2020 general election and seek to mitigate health risks while protecting the election's legitimacy. The report might be of interest to other stakeholders, such as voters themselves and advocates working to support state efforts to prepare for November's election.

This report is part of RAND's Countering Truth Decay initiative, which is focused on restoring the role of facts, data, and analysis in U.S. political and civil discourse and the policymaking process. The original report, *Truth Decay: An Initial Exploration of the Diminishing Role of Facts and Analysis in American Public Life*,[2] laid out a research agenda for studying and developing solutions to the Truth Decay challenge. Truth Decay worsens when individuals lose trust in institutions that could serve as sources of factual information. Legitimate and safe elections can be a first step toward building and maintaining a govern-

---

[1] This report and the research conducted for it are current as of July 27, 2020.

[2] Jennifer Kavanagh and Michael D. Rich, *Truth Decay: An Initial Exploration of the Diminishing Role of Facts and Analysis in American Public Life*, Santa Monica, Calif.: RAND Corporation, RR-2314-RC, 2018.

ment that people trust. This report considers how prepared states are to conduct elections that meet these criteria despite the unique challenges posed by the pandemic.

Funding

Funding for RAND's Countering Truth Decay research initiative is provided by gifts from RAND supporters and income from operations. RAND would like to recognize the Joel and Joanne Mogy Truth Decay Fellowship, established by the Mogys in 2020 to support research on Truth Decay, civics, and democracy. The authors drew from the Mogys' generous gift to fund this project.

Contents

Figures

Tables

Summary

The coronavirus disease 2019 (COVID-19) pandemic has presented a severe threat to state election plans in 2020 for primaries and for the general election. Executive orders that extend access to mail-in ballots and offer other accommodations have provided a stopgap for near-term primary elections, but states still face the challenge of navigating the general election, which will have higher turnout and higher stakes. To conduct an election during the COVID-19 pandemic, states need registration and voting options that minimize direct personal contact and that reduce crowds and common access to high-touch surfaces. Another way to think about preparedness for conducting elections during a pandemic is to consider the flexibility that state election processes afford in terms of where, when, and how voters can get registered and cast votes. Particularly valuable to flexibility in the pandemic context are options that allow for the registration and voting processes to happen remotely or in ways that reduce person-to-person contact. For example, remote voting allows voters to cast a ballot without direct contact with other voters. Early voting can distribute voters across time and locations. States with these options—such as online or automatic registration, remote voting, and early voting—can be considered to have more flexibility on these dimensions and therefore more robustness to the uncertainties associated with COVID-19 and the trajectory of virus spread over the rest of 2020.

The objective of this report is to provide a comprehensive picture of where states stand on these three dimensions of the voting process: voter registration, remote voting, and early voting.[1] (An online database

[1] This report and the research conducted for it are current as of July 27, 2020.

accompanies this report,[2] and a companion report provides an assessment of the access and integrity implications of vote process options.[3]) This picture can be used by state legislatures and election officials to help protect the ability of states to conduct safe and secure elections despite the threat posed by COVID-19. We specifically consider how easily states can shift to remote and distributed registration and voting options that minimize person-to-person contact, first by looking at specific policies and processes and then by considering states' overall preparedness across dimensions. We use states' permanent election laws and processes rather than measures put in place only for 2020 through executive order or temporary provision.

Key Findings

- **Registration.** We find that eight states and the District of Columbia have automatic voter registration (AVR), online registration, and same-day registration and are thus well positioned to register new voters safely (without additional person-to-person contact) and to provide voters several options to minimize personal health risk. Six states have none of these provisions; their registration processes are still conducted in person and as opt-in, stand-alone (*separate*) transactions. These states might encounter the greatest challenges if the COVID-19 pandemic continues through the fall.
- **Remote voting.** All but 16 states have a mail-in or absentee option that is open to all eligible voters and does not require an excuse (hereafter referred to as *no-excuse*). States with unrestricted remote voting might face challenges that stem from having higher numbers of mail-in ballots; nonetheless, they have processes in place to conduct elections without person-to-person contact. The 16 states

---

[2] Jennifer Kavanagh, C. Ben Gibson, and Samantha Cherney, *Database of State Voting Laws: Preparing for Elections During a Pandemic,* Santa Monica, Calif.: RAND Corporation, TL-A112-1, 2020.

[3] See Quentin E. Hodgson, Jennifer Kavanagh, Anusree Garg, Edward W. Chan, and Christine Sovak, *Options for Ensuring Safe Elections: Preparing for Elections During a Pandemic,* Santa Monica, Calif.: RAND Corporation, RR-A112-10, 2020.

that require voters to provide an excuse for absentee voting favor in-person voting, which might create social distancing and sanitation challenges. Twelve states require mail-in or absentee ballots to be signed by a witness or notary. In a pandemic context, this creates an additional person-to-person contact that might raise the risk of virus spread. Six states and the District of Columbia have especially flexible remote voting systems that feature a no-excuse mail-in option, have no witness or notary requirement, and let the voter return the ballot postmarked on Election Day. Another 26 states have processes with the first two characteristics but an earlier deadline. At the other end of the spectrum, five states have processes with none of these characteristics. These five states have less flexibility in their ability to shift toward remote processes with less person-to-person contact.

- **Early voting.** Forty states have early voting options. Six of these have a limited early voting option for those with qualifying reasons. Eight states have early voting periods that extend beyond 30 days, and 13 more have early voting periods that last 16–30 days.
- **Across dimensions.** We consider state registration and voting policies across dimensions by looking specifically at which states have AVR, early voting, and no-excuse mail-in options. In nine states, none of these options are available; these states favor in-person voting on Election Day and require that voters take additional active steps to register. These states will also face the largest challenges in shifting to remote and distributed processes if such a move is required. At the other end of the spectrum, 12 states and the District of Columbia (encompassing about one-third of registered voters) have all three policies, making them among those best positioned for conducting an election during pandemic conditions.

Finally, we create aggregate measures that assess states' registration and voting processes for their ability to shift to remote and distributed options across policies and dimensions. The results are shown in Figure S.1 and Table S.1. States with the lowest rankings have the least flexibility to shift to remote processes and reduce person-to-person contact. With one exception, these states have in-person,

Figure S.1
Flexibility for Pandemic Preparedness Across Dimensions

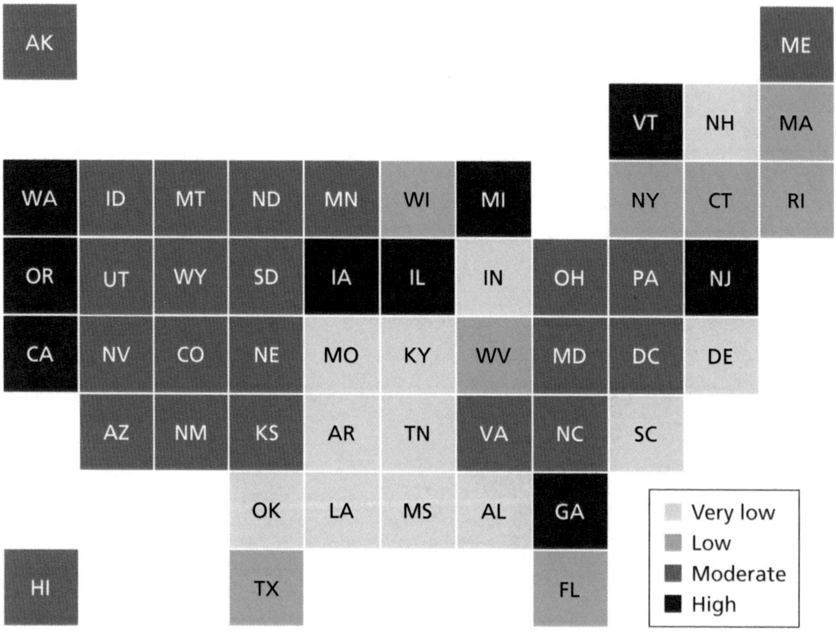

separate-transaction registration processes, excuse-required remote voting, and no early voting. About 25 million registered voters live in these states. States with the highest rankings have the most flexibility on these three policies and are thus perhaps the best situated to deal with the challenges of conducting elections during a pandemic. About 47 million registered voters live in these states. Both the most- and least-flexible groups of states are diverse in terms of size and geographic location. Many states that favor in-person processes and voting on Election Day are in the South; some are in the Northeast, such as Delaware; but very few are in the Western half of the country. Several states with more flexibility for remote processes and early voting are in the West; others are in the Midwest and Northeast. Finally, it is worth noting that a number of states have already taken steps to temporarily shift their voting procedures to incorporate elements of flexibility identified here, including relaxing the excuse requirement for absentee voting and removing the notarization requirement. However, these

Table S.1
States by Flexibility for Pandemic Preparedness

High	Moderate	Low	Very Low
California	Alaska	Connecticut	Alabama
Georgia	Arizona	Florida	Arkansas
Illinois	Colorado	Massachusetts	Delaware
Iowa	District of Columbia	New York	Indiana
Michigan	Idaho	Rhode Island	Kentucky
New Jersey	Hawaii	Texas	Louisiana
Oregon	Kansas	West Virginia	Mississippi
Vermont	Maine	Wisconsin	Missouri
Washington	Maryland		New Hampshire
	Minnesota		Oklahoma
	Montana		South Carolina
	Nebraska		Tennessee
	Nevada		
	New Mexico		
	North Carolina		
	North Dakota		
	Ohio		
	Pennsylvania		
	South Dakota		
	Utah		
	Virginia		
	Wyoming		

temporary changes might not prepare states for future pandemic-like events or similarly disruptive situations.

Acknowledgments

The authors appreciate the support of Michael D. Rich, Terrence Kelly, Henry H. Willis, Jordan R. Fischbach, Erica Robles, and Steph Bingley. They are also grateful for feedback from their reviewers: Scott Bates, Christopher Deluzio, Brian Michael Jenkins, Juliette Kayyem, Geoffrey McGovern, Andrew M. Parker, Michael S. Pollard, and James A. Thomson. Their contributions significantly improved the report. The authors also thank Arwen Bicknell for her excellent editing assistance. Christine Sovak and Kristin Meadows helped with graphics.

CHAPTER ONE

Introduction

As the COVID-19 pandemic triggered the shutdown of businesses, schools, and sports leagues across the United States in March 2020, civic activities were not spared. The shutdown presented a severe and nearly crippling threat to many states' plans to hold primary elections during the spring. Elections are conducted in most states by bringing large groups of people together, often in small spaces, to use shared machines to cast votes. In many counties, the process involves waiting in lines, interacting with "high-touch" surfaces, and having extended close contact with others. But all of these activities were off limits starting in mid-March, when public health experts warned Americans to stay home, avoid interacting with other people (especially in closed spaces), and refrain from touching surfaces that might have been touched by others. The resulting threefold challenge for election officials was significant:

- Conduct secure elections.
- Protect voters from the public health risks of COVID-19 while ensuring that all registered voters can cast a ballot.
- Protect *election integrity* (meaning that the process is free from fraud and guarantees voter privacy).

This unprecedented situation forced many states to delay primary elections. Others changed their processes.[1] Some states—such as Con-

[1] This report and the research conducted for it are current as of July 27, 2020.

necticut, New Hampshire, and New Jersey[2]—used Executive Orders to expand access to absentee ballots for eligible voters or extended absentee ballot deadlines to provide eligible voters more time to submit their ballots.

Although Executive Orders have provided a short-term stopgap for primary elections, states still need to navigate the November 2020 general election, which will have higher turnout and higher stakes. State officials face several challenges in planning for November. First, the fundamental uncertainty about the trajectory of COVID-19 means that states cannot be sure what conditions will look like in November. Epidemiological models that project the spread of the disease vary, but most predict that the United States will continue to face the risk of spikes in COVID-19 cases at least into 2021 and possibly beyond.[3] Some states might decide that shifting to a universal practice of mailing in ballots (*vote-by-mail*) is a safe option to hedge against this uncertainty, but political and legal considerations and resource constraints might hinder some states in implementing such a change in time for November (even if they want to pursue this option). There are costs associated with increasing the security of in-person voting or building the capacity to process larger numbers of mail-in ballots, and analysis indicates that states lack the funds needed to adequately prepare for such changes.[4] There is also the

---

[2] "Governor Lamont Signs Executive Order Allowing All Eligible Connecticut Residents to Vote Absentee in August 11 Primary Elections," Office of Governor Ned Lamont, press release, May 20, 2020; Colby Itkowitz and Amy Gardner, "New Hampshire Governor to Allow Absentee Voting in November Because of Coronavirus Outbreak," *Washington Post*, April 9, 2020; New Jersey Executive Order 105, March 9, 2020.

[3] Stephen M. Kissler, Christine Tedijanto, Edward Goldstein, Yonatan H. Grad, and Marc Lipsitch, "Projecting the Transmission Dynamics of SARS-CoV-2 Through the Post-Pandemic Period," *Science*, Vol. 368, No. 6493, 2020; Christopher Brito, "CDC Director Says Potentially Worse Second Wave of Coronavirus Could Come Along with Flu Season," CBS News, April 23, 2020. See also Kristine A. Moore, Marc Lipsitch, John M. Barry, and Michael T. Osterholm, *COVID-19: The CIDRAP Viewpoint*, Part 1, *The Future of the COVID-19 Pandemic: Lessons Learned from Pandemic Influenza*, Minneapolis, Minn.: Center for Infectious Disease Research and Policy, University of Minnesota, April 30, 2020.

[4] For example, see Lawrence Norden, Edgardo Cortés, Elizabeth Howard, Derek Tisler, and Gowri Ramachandran, *Estimated Costs of COVID-19 Election Resiliency Measures*, New York: Brennan Center for Justice, April 18, 2020; and Alexa Corse, "Voting by Mail to Face Biggest Test Since Pandemic Started," *Wall Street Journal*, June 1, 2020.

question of time: Changes to voting procedures might require changes to legal codes—or at least to state policies and regulations. Such changes can be time-consuming to draft, debate, revise, and implement, even if they do not face political or legal challenges.

For all these reasons, states are starting to examine and modify their election laws and procedures although the election is still several months away. To conduct an election during the COVID-19 pandemic, states need registration and voting options that diverge from the traditional model. Voter registration is essential to conducting elections and might require person-to-person contact at a registrar's office or a voter registration drive. With many offices closed and registration drives and events canceled, states that automatically register voters or that provide online registration options might be better equipped than those that do not. Same-day registration (on Election Day) also might be useful because only one in-person interaction is required, but the process has drawbacks: Voters and poll workers will spend more time in contact with others, and the number of voters who can access a given polling place in a given period might be curtailed.

Voting processes also must minimize direct personal contact and reduce crowds and common access to high-touch surfaces. Vote by mail and early voting are alternatives that spread out the voting period—and the voters themselves—over more days and locations. States vary in the access they provide to voters regarding these two options. For instance, although all states have some sort of absentee voting system that allows for remote voting, some states allow only voters who have qualifying excuses to vote remotely (hereafter referred to as *excuse-required absentee*), meaning that remote voting is open to only some voters. Other states allow mail-in voting for all eligible voters (which covers both no-excuse absentee and mail-in; for simplicity we refer to this as *no-excuse mail-in voting*).

Another way to think about preparedness for conducting elections during a pandemic is to consider the flexibility that a state's election processes afford in terms of where, when, and how voters can get registered and cast votes. Particularly valuable to flexibility in the pandemic context are options that allow for the registration and voting process to happen remotely or in ways that reduce person-to-person contact. States with more options for registration, remote voting, and early voting can be considered to have more flexibility on these dimensions and therefore more robustness in their voting systems to the uncertainties associated with COVID-19. Table 1.1 outlines how flexibility and preparedness map across the three dimensions considered in this report.

It is important to note that policies that promote flexibility and preparedness for a pandemic also have other implications, especially for access and integrity. Processes that expand remote registration, remote voting, or early voting might make it easier for people to vote. In theory, such policies as early voting and remote voting should increase access, but existing research is mixed on whether these provisions significantly affect turnout or simply make the process more convenient for voters who would have voted anyway. Most research suggests that early voting has only a small effect on aggregate turnout.[5] The effect for vote-by-mail seems more sizable but, again, is strongest

Table 1.1
Three Dimensions of Preparedness for Elections During COVID-19 Conditions

Process	Less Flexible	More Flexible
Registration	• In-person registration • Advance registration	• AVR • Online registration • Same-day registration
Remote voting	• Excuse-required absentee • Early due dates for absentee ballots • Notary or witness signature required on ballot	• No-excuse absentee or mail-in option • Universal vote-by-mail • Later deadlines for absentee ballots • Witnesses not needed for voter verification
Early voting	• Early voting limited or prohibited	• Early voting (for extended periods)

NOTES: Our assessment of preparedness is determined by the extent to which an option reduces person-to-person contact. Note that the options here could have different implications for integrity and access, but we focus primarily on preparedness for COVID-19 conditions.

[5] Paul Gronke, Eva Galanes-Rosenbaum, and Peter A. Miller, "Early Voting and Turnout," *PS: Political Science & Politics*, Vol. 40, No. 4, 2007; Robert M. Stein, "Introduction: Early Voting," *Public Opinion Quarterly*, Vol. 62, No. 1, 1998.

for those already inclined to vote. Moreover, the effects of vote-by-mail on turnout have been found to be most limited for high-stakes elections, including presidential contests.[6] Such processes as AVR have also been associated with a small increase in turnout.[7]

At the same time, measures that provide flexibility and can support preparedness for voting during a pandemic also might raise concerns about integrity and fraud. This is especially true of remote voting methods, which critics argue could be more susceptible to violations of election integrity (such as noneligible voters casting ballots, voters casting multiple ballots, or voters who are influenced or coerced to vote a certain way). Although threats to election integrity should be taken seriously, research and analysis of this topic indicate that instances of such fraud are very low.[8] It is true that documented cases of fraud are slightly more common with remote voting than with in-person voting (although they are still minuscule); on the whole, however, policy changes that make registration and voting easier for eligible voters have not resulted in increased incidences of fraud. Furthermore, provisions that are currently in place, such as signature matching, appear to be sufficient to maintain the integrity of the mail-in process.[9]

There is a separate question of whether access or fraud considerations might be fundamentally different under pandemic conditions. Considering questions of access, it seems possible that the benefits of providing at least AVR and remote voting would be amplified by a

---

[6] Jeffrey A. Karp and Susan A. Banducci, "Going Postal: How All-Mail Elections Influence Turnout," *Political Behavior*, Vol. 22, No. 3, 2000; Priscilla L. Southwell and Justin I. Burchett, "The Effect of All-Mail Elections on Voter Turnout," *American Politics Quarterly*, Vol. 28, No. 1, 2000.

[7] Daniel P. Franklin and Eric E. Grier, "Effects of Motor Voter Legislation: Voter Turnout, Registration, and Partisan Advantage in the 1992 Presidential Election," *American Politics Quarterly*, Vol. 25, No. 1, 1997.

[8] Robert M. Stein, *The Incidence and Detection of Ineligible Voting*, paper presented at the American Political Science Association 2013 annual meeting, 2013; Sharad Goel, Marc Meredith, Michael Morse, David Rothschild, and Houshmand Shirani-Mehr, "One Person, One Vote: Estimating the Prevalence of Double Voting in U.S. Presidential Elections," *American Political Science Review*, Vol. 114, No. 2, May 2020; Lori Minnite and David Callahan, *Securing the Vote*, New York: Demos, 2003.

[9] Stein, 2013; Goel et al., 2020; Minnite and Callahan, 2003.

pandemic, which makes it harder and more dangerous for people to gather in person. This would be especially true if states had to reduce the number or capacity of polling locations because of pandemic conditions. On the issue of integrity, some critics suggest that an increase in the volume of mail-in ballots could pose a threat to election integrity by overwhelming state officials, creating new opportunities for fraud, or making such processes as signature matching harder to implement. There is no real evidence that mail-in voting is subject to these threats, so it seems unlikely that the pandemic itself raises the risk of fraud in a meaningful way.[10]

In this report, we do not assess the access and integrity implications of each vote process option. (Our companion report addresses these issues in detail.[11]) Instead, we focus on the extent to which a given process or policy allows a state to enable socially distanced or remote registration and voting as a means to support pandemic preparedness. (We refer to this as *flexibility* and we focus on this flexibility specifically for the robustness it provides for states seeking to conduct elections under the restrictions of the COVID-19 pandemic.) Flexibility in such voter processes as registration and remote and early voting can be beneficial for pandemic preparedness, but there are several other priorities that a state also must balance when setting election processes. States might choose to accept less flexibility on these dimensions to pursue other priorities. In this report, we do not judge what mix of policies a state should pursue; we merely assess the levels of flexibility that states have and the implications for their abilities to pivot quickly to meet the demands of the pandemic. Given how little time states have before the November election, states that already have flexibility

---

[10] Amber Phillips, "Examining the Arguments Against Voting by Mail," *Washington Post*, May 20, 2020. In addition to access and integrity, state officials might wish to consider other factors. For example, there are logistical questions about the time it takes to count and verify a larger number of mail-in ballots. Another issue might be the ability of election officials to audit election results if needed, a process that might be easier with paper ballots than with electronically cast ones. We do not consider these issues in detail.

[11] Quentin E. Hodgson, Jennifer Kavanagh, Anusree Garg, Edward W. Chan, and Christine Sovak, *Options for Ensuring Safe Elections: Preparing for Elections During a Pandemic*, Santa Monica, Calif.: RAND Corporation, RR-A112-10, 2020.

in their registration and voting processes might have an advantage in preparing to conduct elections under the current pandemic conditions.

The objective of this report (and the online database that accompanies it)[12] is to provide a comprehensive picture of where states stand on three dimensions of the voting process—voter registration, remote voting, and early voting—that protect the ability of states to conduct elections without risk to the physical safety of voters while preserving both voter access and election integrity. First, we consider the registration process, especially the availability of automatic, online, and same-day registration. Second, we explore remote voting methods offered in each state. Although some states consider vote-by-mail to be the default option, other states have significant restrictions regarding who can vote in a way other than in person on Election Day. Third, we look at early voting options. In addition to the varying availability of early voting, states also differ in how long early voting locations are open and how many locations are available. We use states' permanent election laws and processes but do not use measures put in place only for 2020 through executive order or temporary provision. However, we do discuss temporary provisions already in place for the November general election in the concluding chapter.

Finally, we look at the overlap of these policies across states and explore which states use which sets of policies, what the most-common combinations of policies seem to be, and what outliers exist. We also consider the geography of these patterns, looking at how the use of different policies or sets of policies is spread out across the United States.[13] We use these comparisons specifically to assess variation in state preparedness along the dimensions outlined in Table 1.1.

---

[12] Jennifer Kavanagh, C. Ben Gibson, and Samantha Cherney, *Database of State Voting Laws: Preparing for Elections During a Pandemic,* Santa Monica, Calif.: RAND Corporation, TL-A112-1, 2020.

[13] The data used for this report were collected from a variety of sources, including the National Association of Secretaries of State, the National Association of State Election Directors, the Election Assistance Commission, Daily Kos, and the National Conference of State Legislatures. In addition to reviewing and comparing across these sources, we also reviewed state statutes. We reached out directly to state and county elections departments for clarifications as needed.

CHAPTER TWO

Registration

Registration is the first step for any voter seeking to cast a ballot. Historically, this activity has been conducted in person at a voter registration drive or a registrar's office. Voter registrations tend to increase substantially in a presidential election year, but the advent of COVID-19 has led to a drop in registration in many states.[1] Voter registration presents a few specific challenges related to COVID-19. First, if voter registration is an in-person process at, for example, a registrar's office, it creates an additional interpersonal interaction with risk of virus spread. Many local government offices are closed because of COVID-19 shutdowns, and this creates yet another challenge to voters seeking to register. The current situation also has led to the cancellation of many voter registration drives and other events where such drives might occur, and it has limited the efforts of groups that provide convenient registration options (such as registering voters at farmers markets or outside subway stops).

There is no single solution to address these challenges, but there are several mitigations that states can consider. One approach is to combine voter registration with another in-person transaction by shifting to an AVR process (for example, as part of the identification processes performed by the Department of Motor Vehicles [DMV] or other local agencies).[2] This approach limits

1 Michael Wines, "Covid-19 Changed How We Vote. It Could Also Change Who Votes," *New York Times*, June 14, 2020.

2 National Conference of State Legislatures, "Automatic Voter Registration," webpage, April 14, 2020c.

the number of in-person contacts (from two to one), but some person-to-person contact is still likely needed. Similarly, states that offer same-day voter registration may offset some risk associated with the COVID-19 pandemic by reducing in-person transactions to just one, but this option requires a voter to spend additional time at a polling place to complete the registration process before voting. Online registration, in contrast, does not require person-to-person contact, but there may be other obstacles that make this option infeasible during a pandemic for some portion of the electorate, especially access to reliable internet or other required technology. Neither challenge is pandemic-specific, but both are exacerbated by the pandemic, when libraries and other places that offer public access may be closed or unsafe. Table 2.1 outlines the policy space that we consider in this chapter. It is also worth noting that North Dakota does not require voter registration: A person is eligible to vote provided they show the required identification, such as a driver's license, identification card, tribal government identification, or long-term care identification with a North Dakota mailing address.[3]

Automatic Voter Registration

Fourteen states and the District of Columbia have AVR,[4] many through DMV locations. Other sites where AVR can take place are health benefit exchanges, local departments of social services, and other designated state offices; typically, the state Secretary of State determines which offices can be sites for AVR. Figure 2.1 identifies states offering AVR as of May 2020. (Note that although we refer to figures as describing states, figures also include the District of Columbia.)

---

[3] Secretary of State North Dakota, "ID Required for Voting," webpage, undated-a.

[4] Maine has passed legislation providing AVR, but this will not take effect until 2022, and West Virginia has passed AVR legislation that will be implemented in 2021 (National Conference of State Legislatures, 2020c).

Table 2.1
Voter Registration Processes

Process	Opt-Out (one transaction)	Opt-In (one transaction)	Opt-In (separate transaction)
In-person	AVR	Same-day registration	Registrar's office
Remote	(No specific registration option)	(No specific registration option)	Online voting

NOTE: Gray cells indicate processes that are more flexible as determined by our framework.

Figure 2.1
States With and Without AVR

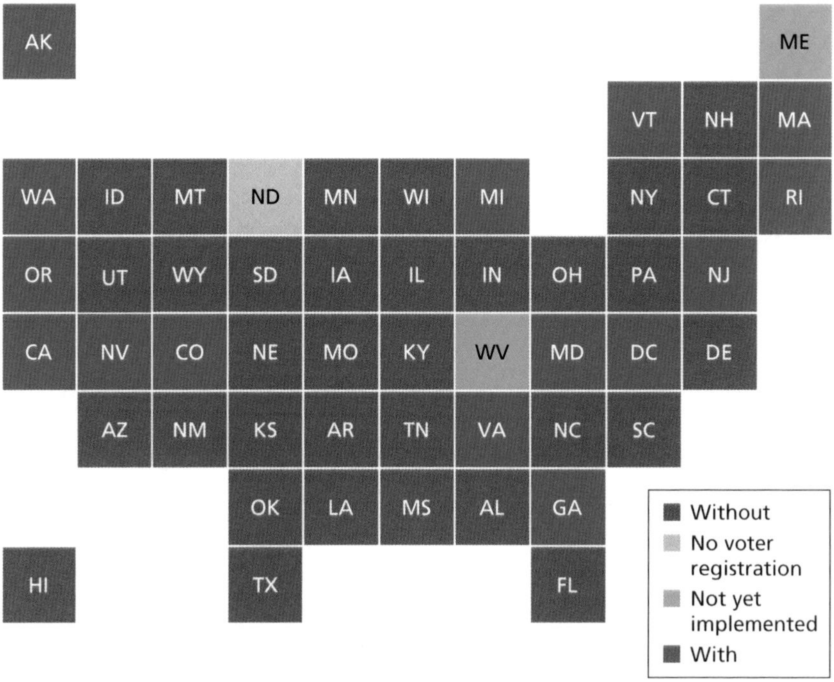

SOURCE: National Conference of State Legislatures, 2020c.
NOTE: Although we refer to states, all figures resembling this one also include the District of Columbia.

There are two main approaches to AVR:[5]

- Some states mail postcards to eligible voters after their qualifying transactions (at the DMV or other location) letting them know that they will be registered to vote unless they opt out by completing and returning a signed form (*preregistration mail notification*).
- In other states, individuals are told at the DMV or other agency that their information will be used to register them to vote unless they explicitly decline (*point-of-service opt-out*).

Most states with AVR use a point-of-service opt-out process, but there are exceptions. Alaska uses a preregistration mail notification method through its Permanent Fund Dividend.[6] Table 2.2 provides information on the distribution of states across these categories.[7]

In addition, there are several states that combine registration with another transaction, as is the case for AVR, but rather than asking individuals to opt out if they do not want to be registered, potential voters have to opt in to be registered. Connecticut, Illinois, Pennsylvania, and

Table 2.2
AVR Methods, by Number of States

Type of AVR	Number of States
Point-of-service opt-out	11 (California, Georgia, Maryland, Massachusetts, Michigan, Nevada, New Jersey, Rhode Island, Vermont, Virginia, and Washington) and the District of Columbia[a]
Preregistration mail notification	3 (Alaska, Colorado, and Oregon)

SOURCE: National Conference of State Legislatures, 2020c.

[a] Maine and West Virginia have plans for this procedure but have not yet implemented them.

---

[5] National Conference of State Legislatures, 2020c.

[6] National Conference of State Legislatures, 2020c.

[7] Throughout this report, we list the primary source of information for tables and maps, but we have also verified all information using the individual state laws. These can be found in the online database that is a companion to this report. See Kavanagh, Gibson, and Cherney, 2020.

Utah provide opt-in registration at the DMV. New Mexico has passed legislation to allow point-of-service opt-in registration, but this has not been implemented.[8]

Same-Day Registration

Another consideration for voting during a pandemic is the availability of same-day registration (on Election Day). Voters choosing to register on the day of the election would have to do so in person, requiring face-to-face contact—but only one transaction would occur, instead of two. Twenty states and the District of Columbia have same-day registration on Election Day. New Mexico has passed same-day election registration legislation but has not implemented it. North Carolina offers same-day registration during the early voting period. As noted at the beginning of this chapter, North Dakota does not have voter registration, but the process for establishing eligibility at the polling place is similar to same-day registration.[9] Figure 2.2 shows the geographic distribution of same-day registration across states.[10]

Next, we consider states that have both automatic registration and same-day registration, thus seeming to offer voters more flexibility in terms of registering to vote.[11] By autumn 2020, eight states and the

---

[8] Brennan Center for Justice, "Policy Differences of Automatic Voter Registration," expert brief, January 17, 2020.

[9] Secretary of State North Dakota, "When Do Eligible Voters Register for an Election?" webpage, undated-b.

[10] States vary in their registration deadlines for the general election. Some states allow for registration up until and including Election Day; others end registration 30 days before the election. Some states offer same-day registration; others have standard registration deadlines some period before the election. For example, Hawaii has a registration deadline of 30 days prior to Election Day for general elections and has same-day registration. Potential voters cannot register in the period between the deadline and Election Day, but they can register in person on Election Day. In some states, such as Connecticut, voters wishing to register and vote on the same day must go to specifically designated locations.

[11] National Conference of State Legislatures, "Same Day Voter Registration," webpage, June 28, 2019a.

Figure 2.2
States With and Without Same-Day Registration

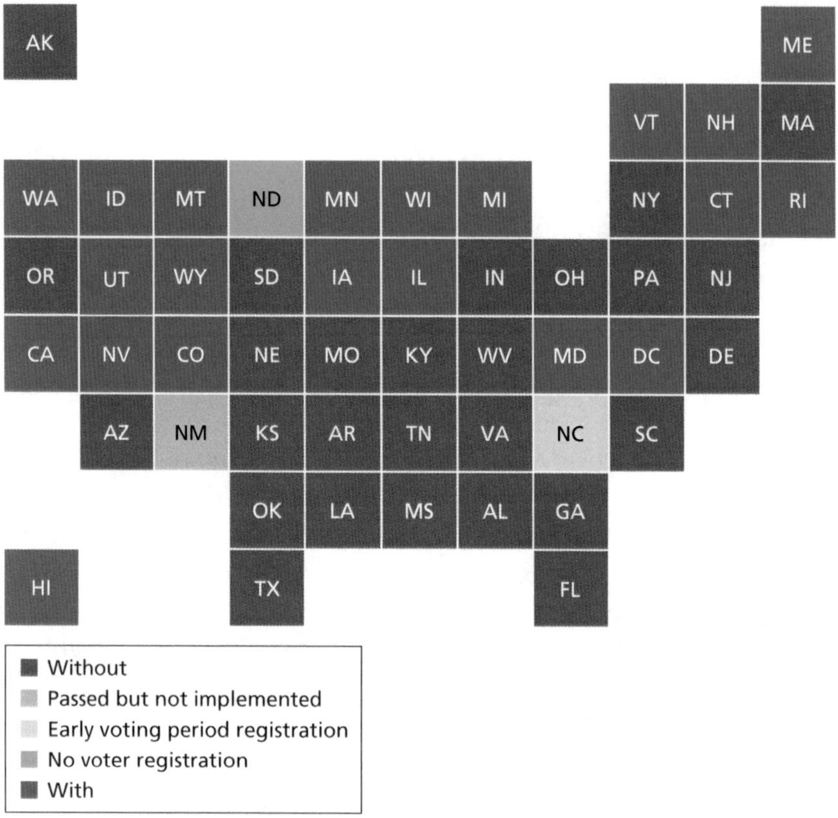

SOURCE: National Conference of State Legislatures, 2019a.
NOTE: Rhode Island allows same-day registration only for presidential elections (thus, it will do so in 2020.)

District of Columbia will offer both AVR and same-day registration. Figure 2.3 shows the geographic distribution of these states.

Online Registration

Finally, online registration is another way that states can reduce in-person interactions for voters and registrants. As of June 2020, 38 states

Figure 2.3
States With and Without Same-Day Registration and AVR

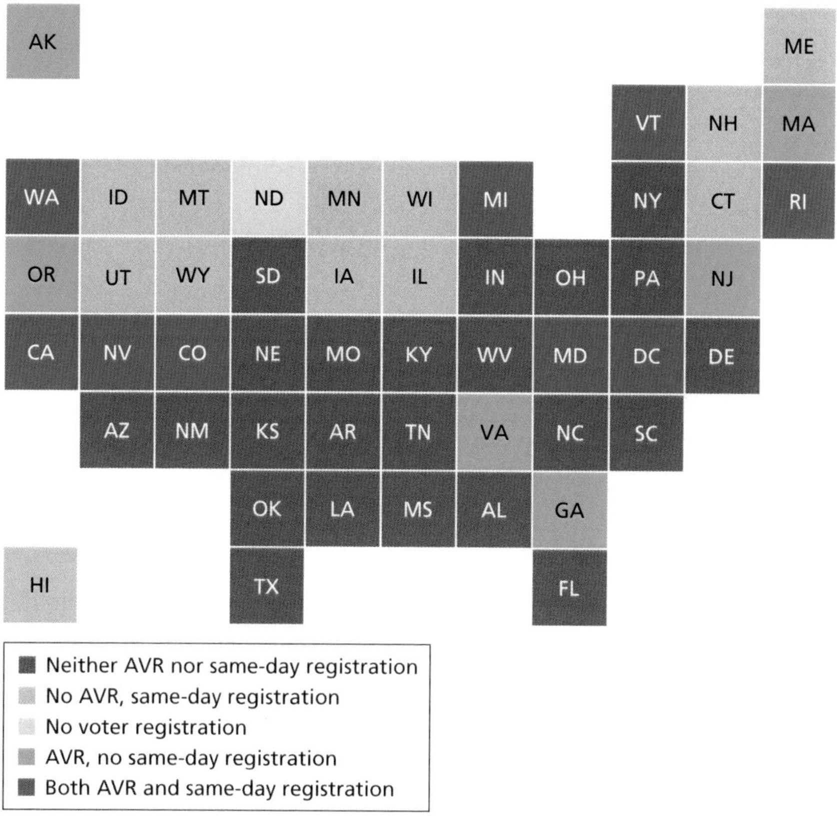

SOURCE: National Conference of State Legislatures, 2019a; National Conference of State Legislatures, 2020c.
NOTE: Rhode Island allows same-day registration only for presidential elections (thus, it will do so in 2020.)

and the District of Columbia offered online registration options, and Oklahoma is phasing in legislation allowing it.[12] Online registration works primarily for those who already have drivers' licenses or official identification cards. Individuals fill out an online form and the infor-

[12] As of June 1, 2020, registered voters could update their registration information online, but new registrations were not yet available online.

Figure 2.4
States with Online Registration and AVR

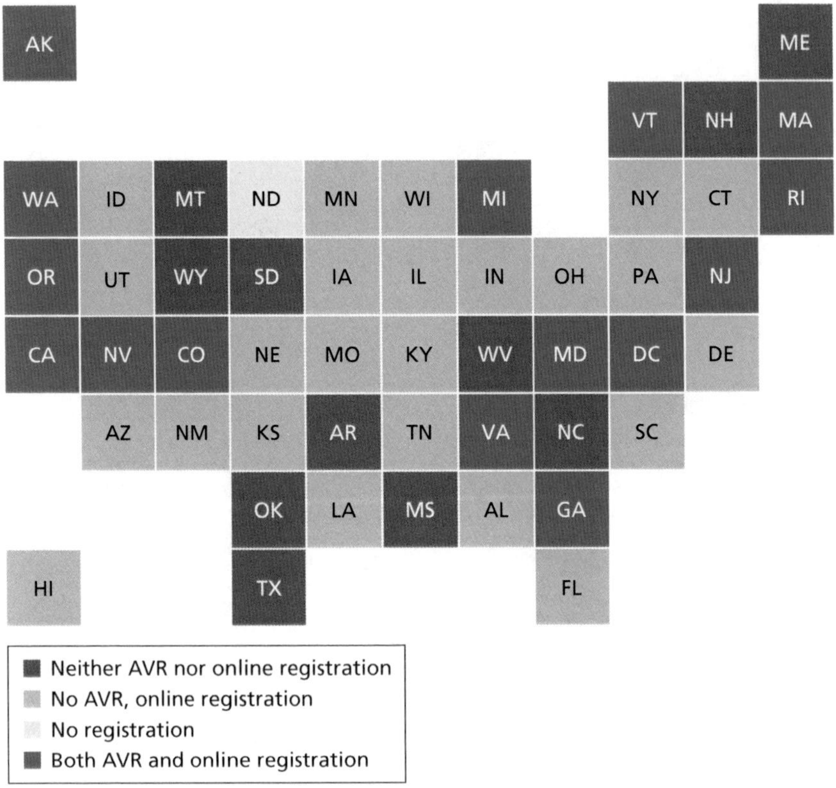

SOURCE: National Conference of State Legislatures, 2020b.

mation provided on it is matched against information they provided when applying for the original license or identification. Online registration is important for states that do not have AVR and for individuals in AVR states who might have completed their "agency transaction" prior to AVR implementation. Figure 2.4 compares states that offer AVR with states that offer online registration.[13] Notably, all states with

[13] National Conference of State Legislatures, "Online Voter Registration," webpage, February 3, 2020b.

AVR also have online registration. But 24 states that do not have AVR do have online registration. Eleven states have neither.

Summary

Although most states have online registration available to those with the right forms of identification, smaller numbers have AVR and/or same-day registration. These three options are not interchangeable; they have different implications for issues of access and election integrity. We focus on flexibility to conduct elections under pandemic conditions that require minimizing person-to-person contact. On that measure, each of these methods has some benefits, but none addresses the problem entirely. Online registration is perhaps the best at mitigating the risk of person-to-person contact, but AVR folds the process into an interaction that would have happened anyway. States with all three options are best-positioned for the situation we are examining.

To assess overall preparedness on the registration dynamic, we can consider which states offer all three (high flexibility on this dimension), two (moderate flexibility), one (low flexibility), or none (no flexibility) of the options outlined in this chapter. This is a simplification—as we noted, these policies are not interchangeable. However, this approach does allow us a simple way to summarize variations across states. Table 2.3 summarizes the number of states by category. Figure 2.5 shows the breakdown geographically.

No state with AVR is in the "low" category in Table 2.3. Seven AVR states are in the moderate category because they do not also have same-day registration. In other words, whether a state has AVR can be a good indicator of its level of flexibility on the registration dimension. As a point of reference, about 79 million registered voters and 169 million Americans live in states that provide high or moderate levels of flexibility on voter registration processes. This represents almost exactly half of both the registered voter population and the U.S. population, leaving the other half more reliant on separate, in-

Table 2.3
Flexibility on Voter Registration Dimension

Flexibility on Voter Registration Processes	Number of States
None	5
Low (one of three options)	21
Moderate (two of three options)	13
High (online, AVR, same-day)	12[a]

NOTE: North Dakota does not require voter registration, so we count it in the "high flexibility" group. Although Connecticut, Illinois, Pennsylvania, and Utah have opt-in processes that are not technically AVR, they do allow for voter registration as part of another transaction, which is the most important aspect from the perspective of our analysis, so we give these states credit for this in the assessment. States that have passed laws but not implemented measures are evaluated based on the law that will prevail in November 2020.

[a] The District of Columbia is included in this number.

person transactions.[14] In contrast, 15 states in the low category offer only the online registration option, and the rest offer only same-day registration. The five states with the lowest level of flexibility (none of these provisions) are Arkansas, Mississippi, Oklahoma, South Dakota, and Texas.

---

[14] Data on population by state were taken from World Population Review, "Number of Registered Voters by State 2020," webpage, undated.

Figure 2.5
States by Flexibility on Voter Registration Processes

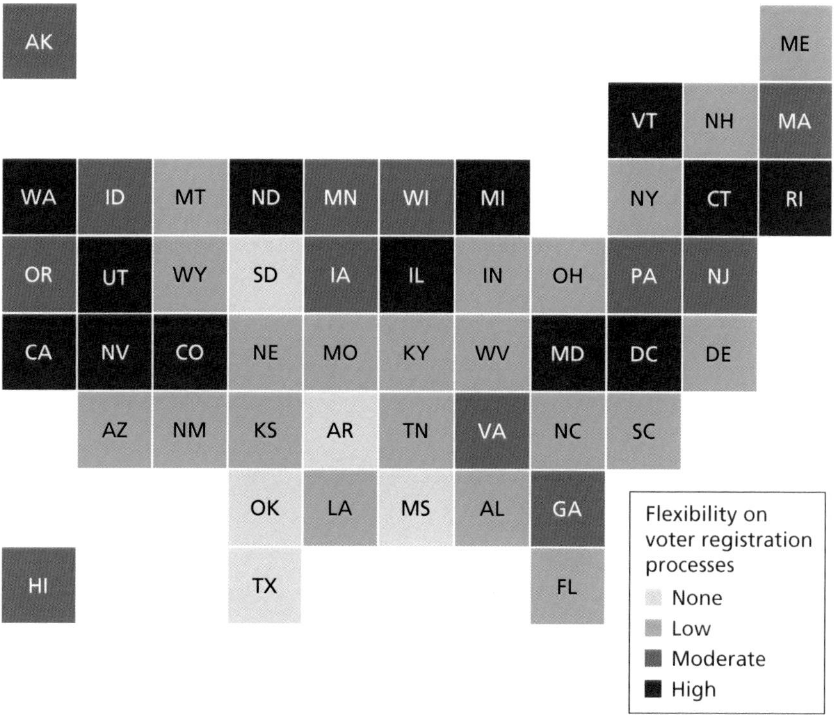

CHAPTER THREE

Remote Voting

The provisions governing remote voting, specifically vote-by-mail and absentee ballots, are another key aspect of state voting law that will shape how elections can be safely conducted in a COVID-19 environment.

Remote Voting Approach

Remote voting options are essential to conducting elections safely during a pandemic because these options allow individuals to vote in ways that reduce or eliminate person-to-person contact. Reduction in interpersonal contact (either by allowing people to vote remotely or by spreading out the process over time) not only reduces the risk of virus spread for or by these individuals; it also reduces the risk to those who do vote in person on Election Day. We consider four main approaches to remote voting:[1]

- **Excuse-required absentee voting:** Absentee ballots are provided only to individuals who have a qualifying excuse. Qualifying reasons can be disabilities or illnesses that prevent voting in person, being out of the state on Election Day, or having work hours that extend across the entire time when the polls are open. To receive a ballot, the individual must request one and provide an excuse.

[1] National Academies of Sciences, Engineering, and Medicine, *Securing the Vote: Protecting American Democracy*, Washington, D.C.: National Academies Press, 2018; National Conference of State Legislatures, "Voting Outside the Polling Place: Absentee, All-Mail and Other Voting at Home Options," webpage, June 9, 2020d.

States vary in the ways that they verify the excuse provided. Most states do not require individuals to provide proof of their qualifying excuse, but all states require voters to attest that the information on their applications is accurate, on penalty of substantial fines or imprisonment. Voters requesting longer-term absentee ballots for medical reasons or because of a disability typically have to provide certification of their medical concern.

- **No-excuse absentee voting:** Any eligible voter can request an absentee ballot and vote remotely. No excuse is needed.
- **Permanent vote-by-mail:** Similar to no-excuse absentee voting, any eligible voter can vote remotely; furthermore, individuals can choose to become permanent vote-by-mail voters and receive a ballot in the mail every election afterward. Most states that provide this option also offer no-excuse absentee voting.
- **Universal vote-by-mail:** Nearly all voting occurs via mail-in ballots that are provided to all registered voters; very limited in-person voting is provided in special circumstances. Ballots can also be returned to specially provided drop-off boxes and do not always require return by mail.

In addition to these four categories, there is one outlier: Pennsylvania has an absentee process that requires an excuse but also a mail-in option that is open to anyone.[2] The mail-in option allows voters to request a mail-in ballot for a full year.[3] Our assessment does not include special classes of voters, such as military voters and Americans living abroad. The Uniformed and Overseas Citizens Absentee Voting Act provides these voters with absentee voting options, including online and by fax, and they often have a later deadline than other absentee

---

[2] Pennsylvania's constitution provides for absentee voting under certain circumstances. The mail-in option was added to absentee voting rather than replacing it to stay in compliance with the state constitution. See Constitution of the Commonwealth of Pennsylvania, Article VII, paragraph 14, "Absentee Voting."

[3] Commonwealth of Pennsylvania, "Voting in Pennsylvania," webpage, undated.

voters. We omit this group because these individuals are already well positioned to vote during a pandemic.[4]

Remote voting has implications outside those directly related to the pandemic. For example, the type of remote voting that a state chooses to implement could have implications for how quickly it is able to finalize election results. States with earlier ballot deadlines or fewer mail-in votes might be better able to finalize results on Election Night; in other states, counting of ballots can extend past Election Night. An assessment of this implication is outside the scope of our report but might be relevant to the considerations of state election officials. Table 3.1 shows the number of states that use each of these four methods; Figure 3.1 shows the geographic distribution of these states. As a point of reference, about 104 million registered voters (about two-thirds of the registered voting population in 2020) live in states with some sort of no-excuse mail-in option.[5]

Table 3.1
Remote Voting Methods, by Number of States

Type of Remote Voting	Number of States
Excuse-required absentee	16
Excuse-required absentee and no-excuse mail-in	1
No-excuse absentee and permanent mail-in	8[a]
No-excuse absentee	21
Universal mail-in (only)	5

SOURCE: National Conference of State Legislatures, 2020d.

NOTES: Rhode Island refers to its remote voting process as vote-by-mail, but the process best approximates what we define here as "no-excuse absentee." The state allows permanent vote-by-mail for those with certified disabilities. See State of Rhode Island Board of Elections, "Mail Ballot," webpage, undated. A number of states have temporarily amended their voting procedures for the November 2020 general election. This table reports the permanent process. We list temporary provisions in Chapter Five.

[a] The District of Columbia is included in this number.

---

[4] U.S. Department of Justice, "The Uniformed and Overseas Citizens Absentee Voting Act," webpage, February 26, 2020.

[5] Data on population by state were taken from World Population Review, undated.

Figure 3.1
States by Remote Voting Method

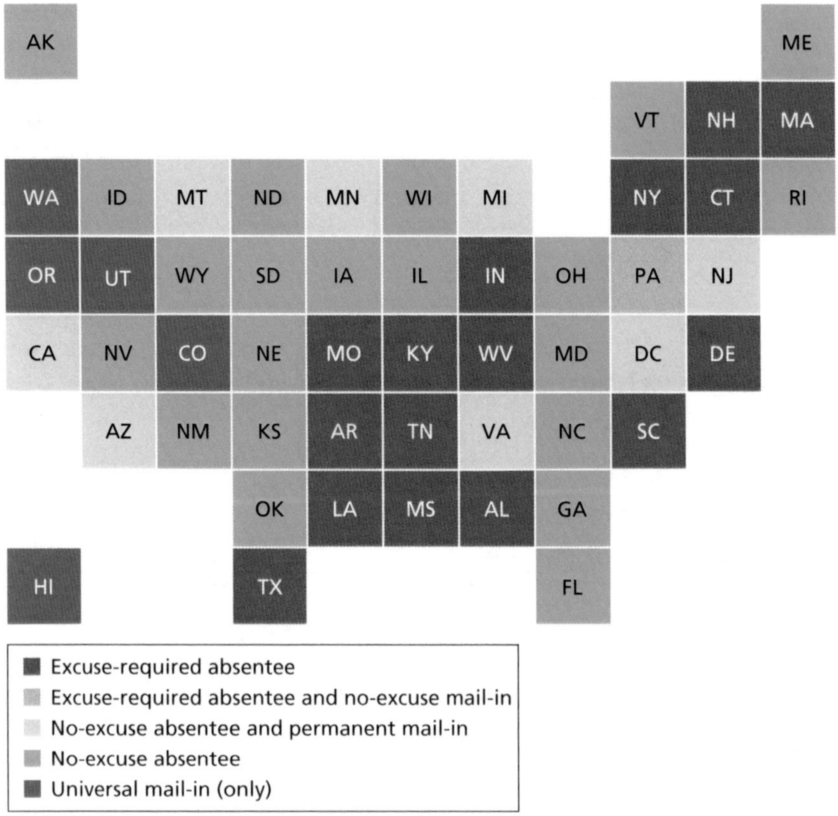

SOURCE: National Conference of State Legislatures, 2020d.

Absentee Ballot Due Dates

Other characteristics of remote voting systems might be relevant to the application of these laws during a pandemic. Due dates of mail-in or absentee ballots vary.[6] Receipt deadlines for mail-in or absentee

---

[6] Another set of deadlines that could affect preparedness are those for requesting absentee ballots. There is limited variation on this dimension, so we do not consider it extensively. Most states set a deadline between 0 and 10 days before the election for absentee applications to be submitted. A handful of cases (most with excuse-required absentee voting), set earlier

ballots are most relevant to pandemic preparedness for cases in which the remote voting process presents challenges or delays as a result of the pandemic. For example, ballots might be mailed to voters late as officials struggle to deal with increasing numbers of mail-in voters or to manage the process with reduced staff. Glitches in the processing of mail-in requests could also cause problems if some voters do not receive their ballots. To guard against these issues, later deadlines (such as allowing voters to postmark their ballots on Election Day rather than requiring receipt on or before that day) might support preparedness.

Table 3.2 and Figure 3.2 show states organized by when absentee or mail ballots are due. About 70 percent have Election Day as the received-by due date. One state, Louisiana, requires that absentee ballots be received by 4:30 p.m. the day before the election. A small number of states require that mailed ballots be postmarked by the day before Election Day. In some cases, these states also allow voters to return ballots to their polling place or a drop box at the registrar's office. Finally, 12 states accept ballots received after the election, provided that they are postmarked by Election Day. In the District of Columbia, ballots must be postmarked by Election Day and received within seven days of the election. Alaska allows voters ten days after the election. West Virginia allows absentee ballots that are received by the day after the election or that are received by the time the Board of Canvassers meets if postmarked by Election Day.[7] This "postmarked by Election Day" deadline provides voters the most time to complete and submit their ballot without having to return it in person.

State governments do have some flexibility under certain circumstances to change the receipt deadline for absentee ballots for a particular election. However, this flexibility varies by state. In 2020, states have achieved varying levels of success in their efforts to change deadlines. In Pennsylvania, Governor Tom Wolf was able to extend the receipt date for jurisdictions that had disaster declarations because of

---

deadlines. Most states also have an emergency provision that allows individuals to request and receive an absentee ballot even after the deadline if they meet required conditions.

[7] National Conference of State Legislatures, "Receipt and Postmark Deadlines for Absentee Ballots," webpage, June 15, 2020e.

Table 3.2
Mail-In Ballot Due Dates

Due Date	Number of States
Before Election Day	1
Postmarked day before Election Day	4
On Election Day	34
Postmarked by Election Day	12[a]

SOURCE: National Conference of State Legislatures, 2020e.

[a] The District of Columbia is included in this number.

Figure 3.2
States by Mail-In Ballot Due Dates

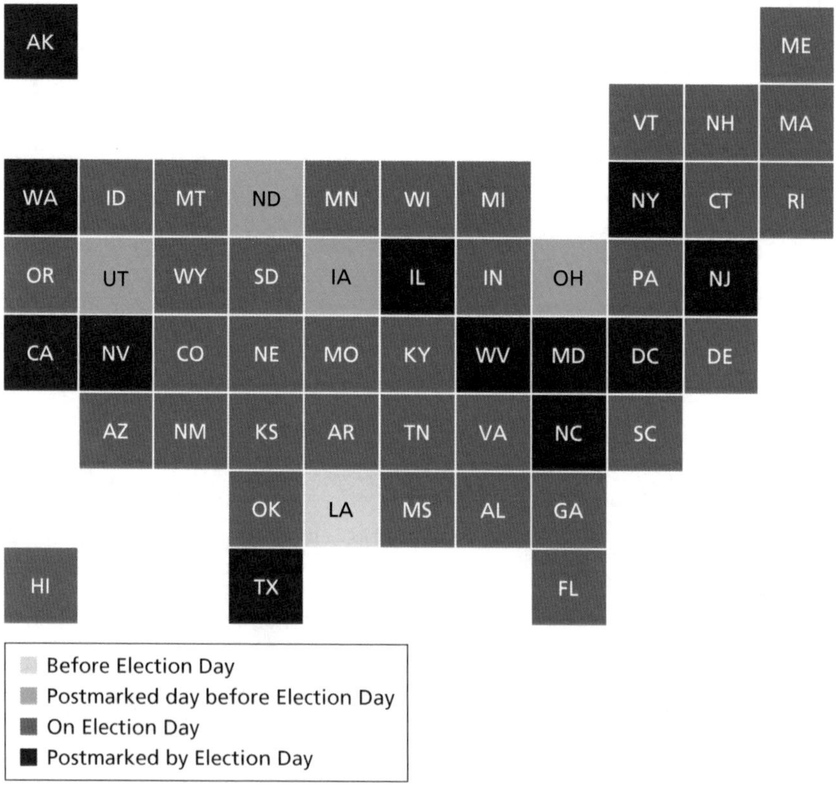

SOURCE: National Conference of State Legislatures, 2020e.

racial justice protests, but a similar effort in Wisconsin in response to the COVID-19 pandemic encountered opposition from the legislature and was ultimately disallowed by the Supreme Court.[8] We can expect that efforts to change deadlines for the November election will vary in success and generate legal challenges.

Verification

Next, we consider how absentee ballots are verified. The level of scrutiny applied to mail-in ballots, in terms of verifying their authenticity, varies by state. States put various requirements into place in different combinations. Those with fewer verification provisions ask voters only to sign a statement or oath on the ballot envelope attesting to its validity and their own eligibility. Other states rely on a manual or automated signature matching process that compares the voter's signature on the ballot with that submitted as part of the registration process. Still other states add a witness or proof-of-identification requirement to the signature match or signed voter statement. The highest bar is set by states requiring that the signed ballot be notarized by a notary public or other eligible official. All these options have different implications for elections conducted during a pandemic. Systems that require notarization do little to minimize in-person interaction and create a transaction that would not happen otherwise. These systems also could encounter logistical challenges if the number of absentee voters rises sharply and exceeds the capacity of notaries. States that require one or more witnesses similarly create additional person-to-person contact. It is possible that such requirements could be met by family members who are already in the voter's household, but if the voter needs to go outside the family, this creates a new risk of virus spread. Signature matching and signed statements do not create new interpersonal contacts, but signature matching systems can be labor intensive (as we will discuss in more detail). This matters if the volume

---

8 "Gov. Wolf Signs Executive Order Extending Mail Ballot Deadline in Six Counties to June 9," Governor Tom Wolf Newsroom, press release, June 1, 2020; Tucker Higgins, "US Supreme Court Sides with GOP in Wisconsin: Absentee Ballots Must Be Sent by Tuesday," CNBC, April 6, 2020.

of absentee ballots increases dramatically. Each of these options also has implications for access and integrity. For instance, systems that require notarization place a high burden on the voter, potentially reducing access, but they are intended to guard against fraud (although evidence of such fraud is limited).[9] We do not tackle these issues in detail; our focus is on preparedness to counter safety concerns. Table 3.3 breaks down the number of states that use each verification approach; Figure 3.3 shows the geographic distribution of those states.[10]

The vast majority of states (60 percent) rely only on signature match. Signature matching can be done electronically or manually. An electronic system is likely quicker and less resource-intensive than matches done by hand, but it might have less ability to detect nuance and make decisions based on small discrepancies that perhaps do not warrant rejection. On the other hand, an electronic approach can be more consistent and easier to audit. Many states use a combination of both methods, first using an electronic scanner and then using manual

Table 3.3
Mail-In Ballot Verification Approaches

Due Date	Number of States
Signed statement	9[a]
Signed statement and witness	4
Signature match	30
Signature matching and witness	4
Signature and notarized affidavit	4

SOURCE: National Conference of State Legislatures, "Verification of Absentee Ballots," webpage, January 21, 2020a.

NOTE: A number of states have temporarily amended their voting procedures for the November 2020 general election. This table reports the permanent process. We list temporary provisions in Chapter Five.

[a] The District of Columbia is included in this number.

---

[9] Elaine Kamarck and Christine Stenglein, "Low Rates of Fraud in Vote-by-Mail States Show the Benefits Outweigh the Risks," Brookings Institution, June 2, 2020.

[10] National Conference of State Legislatures, 2020a; Vote Riders, "Voter ID for Absentee Ballots," webpage, undated.

Figure 3.3
States by Mail-In Ballot Verification Approach

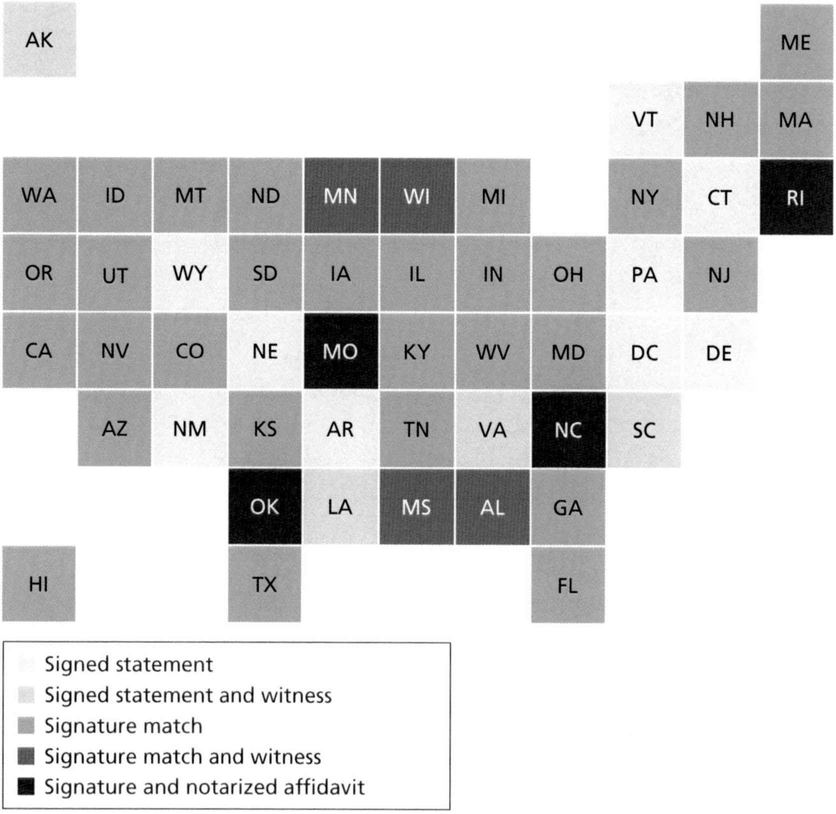

SOURCE: National Conference of State Legislatures, 2020a.
NOTE: North Carolina and Rhode Island require signature matching plus notarization or 2 witnesses. We code these in the "signature and notarized affidavit" category, but note that signature and two witnesses is an alternative in both states.

inspection on ballots that are disputed.[11] The requirements and approach to verifying signatures is publicly available information in all states, but there are variations in how this information is provided to individuals and whether individuals must search for this information on their own.

---

[11] "Rush to Vote-by-Mail Requires Decisions on Signature Verification," Global Newswire, April 23, 2020; Susie Armitage, "Handwriting Disputes Cause Headaches for Some Absentee Voters," Propublica, November 5, 2018.

Some states require a signed statement or signature matching and the signature of an eligible witness: South Carolina requires the signature of a witness; Mississippi requires both a signature matching and a witness. Other states require that the signed ballot be notarized: Oklahoma requires that the signed ballot be notarized; Rhode Island requires a signature matching and either the signature of a notary or of two witnesses. These states might be less prepared for conducting an election under pandemic conditions because they require additional person-to-person contact by the voter, partially offsetting the benefits of having a remote voting option.

A final consideration is that of voter identification requirements. In our review, we identified three states that require the voter to submit some sort of voter identification (such as a copy of a driver's license or state identification card) along with their ballot: Arkansas, Alabama, and Missouri.[12] The voter identification requirement certainly has access and integrity implications but fewer implications for pandemic preparedness. Many states require some proof of identification as part of the absentee or mail-in ballot request process.

Remedies for Discarded Ballots

Finally, we consider ways for voters to verify that mail-in or absentee ballots have been counted and to address cases in which a mailed ballot is found to have been disallowed or discarded. Not all states outline a procedure for the remedy of discarded ballots. Of those that do, some provide affected voters with a notification; others require voters to investigate themselves through an online database or other method. States also vary in the speed of notification and the process they provide for voters to cure the ballot (or address the reason for its rejection). We found that 24 states and the District of Columbia define a process for individuals to seek out information about whether their ballot was accepted. Seven states (Delaware, Maryland, New Hampshire, New Jersey, Oklahoma, Pennsylvania, and West Virginia) require the voter

[12] National Conference of State Legislatures, 2020a; Vote Riders, undated.

to seek out information on ballot status. Among states that provide notification, timing varies from as soon as possible to after Election Day. With the potential for more absentee voters during the COVID-19 pandemic, preparedness is likely enhanced by ensuring that some process is in place allowing voters to verify that their ballot was counted, if only to reduce the number of inquiries and the administrative burden on election officials. It is not clear whether one system is better than another from this preparedness viewpoint, but from an access perspective, a system in which voters are notified directly reduces the burden placed on the voter. Figure 3.4 shows the geographic distribution of states as determined by this aspect of their remote voting system.

States also differ in the options they provide to affected voters—that is, ways that the voter can cure the ballot or address the reason for rejection. In 11 states, election officials are required to address the problem before or on Election Day; in most cases, this is done by providing a replacement ballot or asking the affected individual to vote in person on Election Day.[13] Systems requiring the latter approach create new in-person interactions and negate the benefits of remote voting for the affected individual and are thus less suited for pandemic conditions.

Summary

States vary significantly in their remote voting systems, and those systems vary in how efficiently they might allow elections to be conducted under pandemic conditions. Not only do they vary in terms of the availability of remote voting options, they also vary in terms of how long individuals have to return their ballots, how these ballots are authenticated, and how individuals whose ballots might have been discarded can rectify the situation. The most-prepared states are those with universal vote-by-mail. States with no-excuse absentee and/or no-excuse mail-in options are also well positioned but might need to consider how they will deal with a larger volume of such ballots in the fall. Least prepared are those states with only excuse-required absen-

---

[13] National Conference of State Legislatures, 2020a.

Figure 3.4
States by Remedy Process

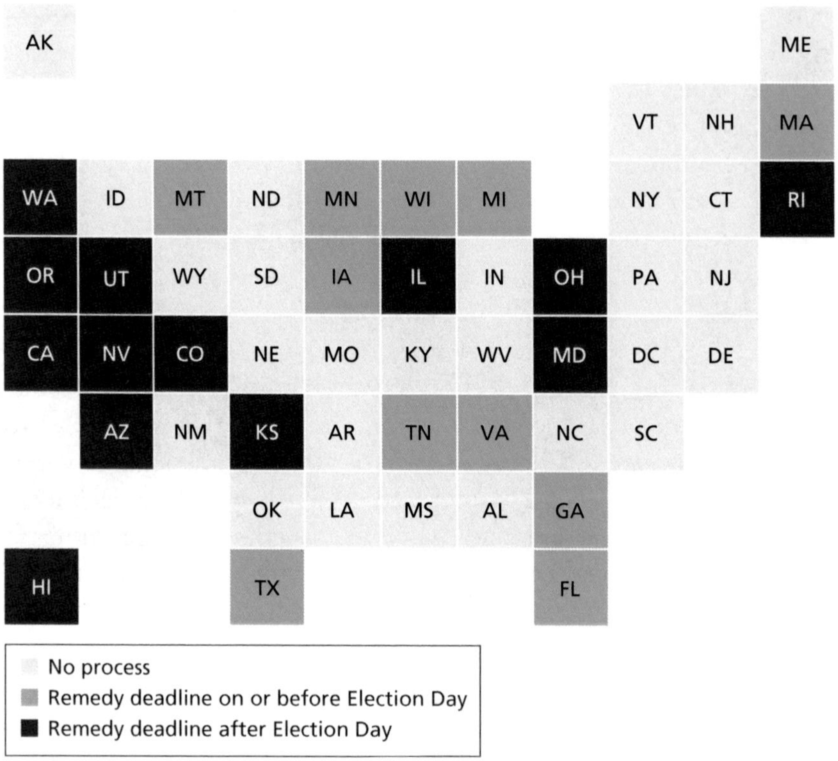

SOURCE: National Conference of State Legislatures, 2020a.

tee options. Other aspects of remote voting also could shape states' preparedness. States with absentee deadlines that allow postmarking on Election Day and those with verification systems that do not rely on witnesses and notaries might be the best positioned to navigate the challenges of conducting an election during a pandemic.

States also vary in the flexibility they demonstrate in their remote voting processes across the characteristics described in this chapter. We consider three characteristics, each coded into yes or no categories: availability of no-excuse vote-by-mail; absentee ballot due dates of postmark by Election Day (the latest deadline in the sample, giving voters the most options for returning their ballots); and verification processes that do not require witnesses or notaries. Our assessment provides each of these characteristics equal weight. Arguably, access to a no-excuse mail-in ballot is the most central provision on this dimension required to conduct safe elections during a pandemic. However, even easy access to such a ballot for eligible voters would have limited value if voters then struggle with finding necessary witnesses or submitting their ballot on time.

Table 3.4 illustrates how many states have all three of these characteristics (no-excuse mail-in option, postmarked on Election Day deadline, and no witness or notary requirement), which we term "high flexibility" on the remote voting dimension; how many have two characteristics (moderate flexibility), how many have one (low flexibility), and how many have none. Again, we use the term *flexibility* here specifically in reference to the state's ability to easily prepare for conducting an election during a pandemic. Figure 3.5 displays the geographic distribution of these states. In each case, high flexibility is useful to the extent that it allows states to easily pivot during the November election and mitigate a variety of risks stemming from the COVID-19 pandemic. We found that only six states and the District of Columbia fall into the high flexibility category (accounting for about 34 million registered voters). Among states in the moderate category, 21 have both a no-excuse mail-in option and a verification method that does not require a witness or notary but have ballot receipt deadlines on or before Election Day. In other words, these states have a high degree of flexibility in their remote

Table 3.4
Flexibility on Remote Voting Dimension

Flexibility	Number of States
None	5
Low (one of three characteristics)	13
Moderate (two of three characteristics)	26
High (no-excuse absentee, postmarked on Election Day, no witness or notary)	7[a]

SOURCE: National Conference of State Legislatures, 2020a.
NOTE: A number of states have temporarily amended their voting procedure for the November 2020 general election. This table is based on permanent voting procedures. We list temporary provisions in Chapter Five.
[a] The District of Columbia is included in this number.

Figure 3.5
States by Flexibility on Remote Voting Dimension

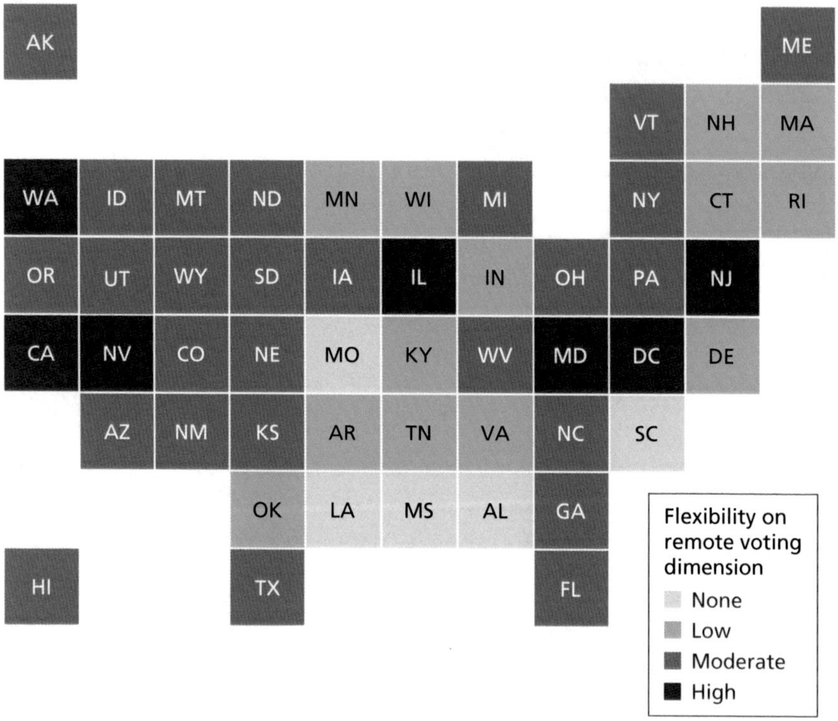

SOURCE: National Conference of State Legislatures, 2020a.

voting process, but the earlier deadline could become a constraint in the event of glitches or challenges. Among states in the low flexibility category, most require excuses for absentee voting. The five states with the least flexibility on the remote voting dimension are Alabama, Louisiana, Mississippi, Missouri, and South Carolina (about 12 million voters).

Overall, almost 64 percent of states (about 112 million registered voters)[14] have moderately to very flexible processes that provide a foundation for conducting elections in the fall. On the other hand, 18 states have limited flexibility and might be less resilient to pandemic-related disruptions.

---

[14] Data on population by state were taken from World Population Review, undated.

CHAPTER FOUR

Early Voting

A final category of election-related legislation worth considering in the context of an election conducted under pandemic conditions is early in-person voting, which is what it sounds like: Voters can submit ballots in person before Election Day.[1] The availability of early voting can help reduce the volume of people voting on Election Day and thus allow social distancing to be implemented more effectively. Early voting also allows more time to disinfect common high-touch surfaces and might ease the implementation of other safety protocols. States that have early voting—especially those that have longer periods for early voting—might be better prepared to conduct an election under pandemic conditions than states that do not have early voting or states that offer early voting only for individuals who have a valid reason for not voting on Election Day (in those states, criteria for early voting are the same as those for excuse-required absentee voting).

First, we consider which states permit early voting. Figure 4.1 shows the geographic distribution of these states. Thirty-nine states and the District of Columbia have some form of early voting, accounting for about 128 million registered voters (or more than 80 percent of registered voters). An additional six states have early voting but only

[1] States that have early voting systems vary in how they execute the early voting process. In some states, early voting operates like Election Day voting, with voters going to a polling place as they would on Election Day. Other states use early in-person absentee voting, which allows voters to fill out an absentee ballot prior to Election Day. We consider both processes together as "early voting" because they have largely the same implications for states conducting elections during a pandemic.

Figure 4.1
States by Early Voting Availability

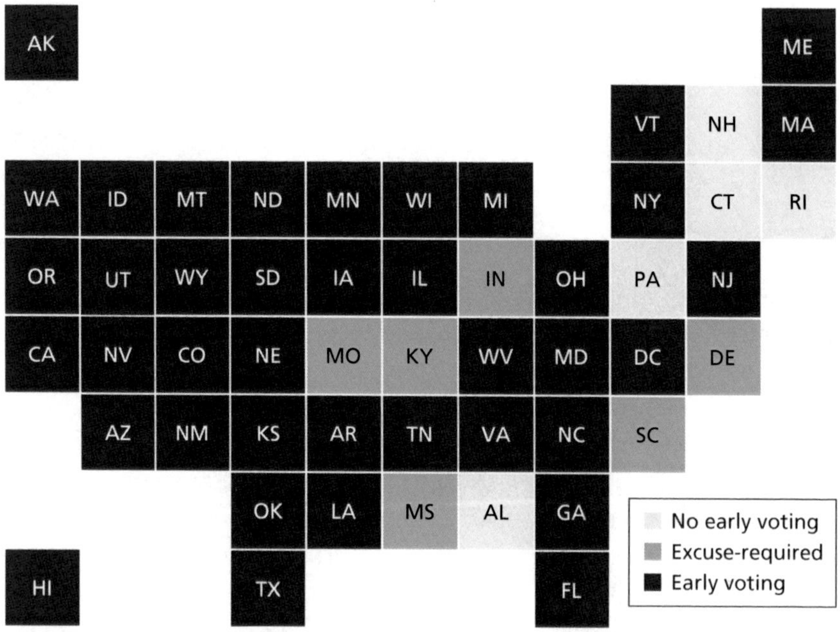

SOURCE: National Conference of State Legislatures, "State Laws Governing Early Voting," webpage, August 2, 2019b.

for those meeting the excuse requirement for absentee voting. In these states, individuals wishing to vote early must have a qualifying excuse for why they cannot vote on Election Day. Seven states have both excuse-required absentee voting and early voting open to anyone. This is an interesting mix of policies: The ability to vote early expands the ability to vote on a day other than Election Day (though not the ability to vote remotely) to a larger group of people than only those meeting a list of valid excuses. We consider these policy combinations in further detail in the next section. Only five states (Alabama, Connecticut, New Hampshire, Pennsylvania, and Rhode Island) had no early voting provisions as of May 25, 2020.[2]

[2] National Conference of State Legislatures, 2019b; Brennan Center for Justice, "Voting Laws Roundup 2020," webpage, undated.

Early Voting Period

The length of time set aside for early voting to occur varies significantly, from 45 days to less than a week. States with longer early voting periods can better reap the crowd-management benefits of early voting because, in theory, they can spread out voters across more days and potentially attract a greater number of individuals to the early voting option. We exclude states that restrict early voting to those with an excuse that enables absentee voting because these states do not take full advantage of the flexibility afforded by early voting. Table 4.1 and Figure 4.2 show the distribution of these states. Even states with similar time frames for early voting vary in terms of the windows provided on those days. For some states, the window extends right up to Election Day. For others, it stops short of Election Day but starts earlier. Some states offer weekend hours; others do not. Some have a minimum time-length requirement for the early voting period, but that period can be lengthened at the discretion of the Secretary of State or other election official.[3]

Number of Early Voting Locations

We find that few states provide explicit guidance on the numbers of locations that must be provided for early voting. In six states, the minimum number is legislated based on a given number per county or on population size. A handful of states set minimum conditions on such aspects as hours that early voting must be offered and offer guidance on locations that are eligible to be early voting polling locations. Most states permit early voting at a variety of different government buildings, such as elections offices and other public facilities. For example, New Mexico requires that early voting be offered at county clerks' offices and at alternative locations determined by the number of voters (for example, counties with 10,000 voters must have one additional location); it also regulates the hours of early voting sites, noting that locations must be open eight consecutive hours, open no earlier than 7 a.m., and close no

---

3 National Conference of State Legislatures, 2019b.

Table 4.1
Duration of Early Voting Period

Number of Early Vote Days	Number of States
1–15 days	19[a]
16–30 days	13
31–45 days	8

SOURCE: National Conference of State Legislatures, 2019b.

[a] The District of Columbia is included in this number.

Figure 4.2
States by Available Early Voting Period

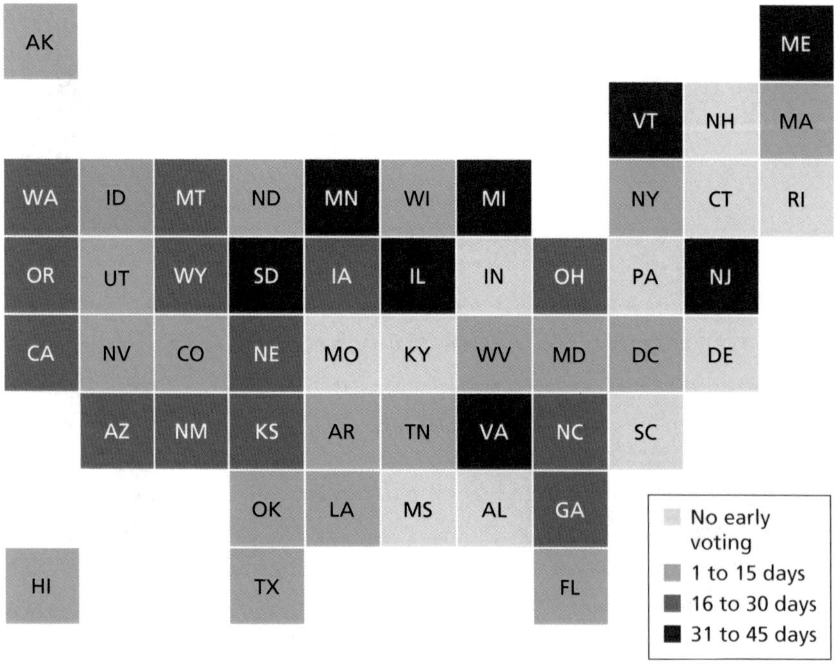

SOURCE: National Conference of State Legislatures, 2019b.
NOTE: "No early voting" includes states with early voting options that are restricted to those with qualifying excuses.

Table 4.2
Polling Location Regulations

Regulations on Number of Polling Locations	Number of States
Rules on minimum only	6
Rules on maximum only	0
Rules on both	1

later than 9 p.m. Alternative locations might close Sunday, Monday, or both. Maryland, in contrast, provides guidance only on the minimum and maximum numbers of locations.[4] Table 4.2 shows states organized by whether they define a minimum or maximum standard of polling locations. From the perspective of conducting an election during a pandemic, more locations are preferable: A large number of locations for early voting allows voters to spread out more and improve social distancing.

Summary

States vary in the availability of early voting as an option, the duration of the period for early voting, and the number of locations available. To assess preparedness on this dimension, we focus on the first two characteristics; the information available on the third is more limited. The eight states (24.5 million registered voters) that have the longest periods for early voting (31–45 days) can be considered among the most flexible and likely the best prepared to conduct an election under pandemic conditions, followed by the 13 states (47 million registered voters) that have early voting periods of 16–30 days. States without any early voting or with early voting restrictions are least prepared. Table 4.3 repeats these categories of states organized by level of flexibility, and Figure 4.3 shows their geographic distribution.[5]

In the next chapter, we consider how the three areas of preparedness considered thus far (voter registration, remote voting, and early voting) overlap and which states appear to have the most-flexible voting policies

---

[4] National Conference of State Legislatures, 2019b.

[5] Data on population by state were taken from World Population Review, undated.

Table 4.3
Flexibility on Early Voting Dimension

Number of Early Vote Days	Number of States
No or restricted early vote	11
Low (early vote, short early vote period)	19[a]
Moderate (early vote, medium early vote period)	13
High (early vote, long early vote period)	8

[a] The District of Columbia is included in this number.

Figure 4.3
States by Flexibility on Early Voting

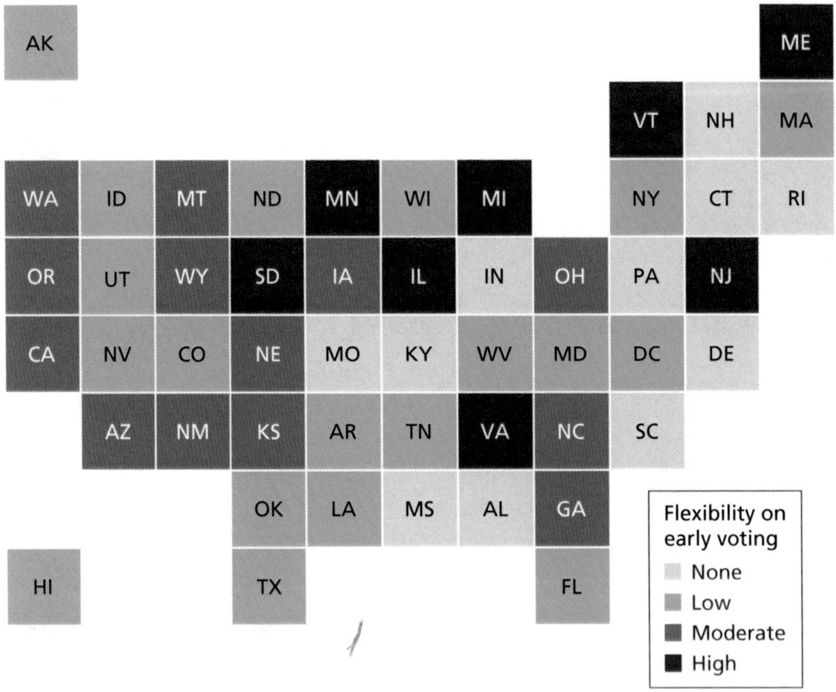

across all three dimensions, making them better prepared for and resilient to shocks.

CHAPTER FIVE

State Types

In this chapter, we consider how states vary across all three dimensions of the voting process considered in this report. We do this by using specific pieces of the state process and relying on the aggregated measures of flexibility that we developed and discussed in previous chapters. First, we consider the overlap of three specific types of policies: AVR, no-excuse mail-in option (absentee or mail vote), and early voting. We choose AVR as the dimension of registration to focus on because, as noted previously, states with AVR are also likely to have several of the other dimensions of flexibility on registration. Second, we compare states across dimensions in terms of their flexibility to navigate conducting an election under pandemic conditions using our summary indicators.

Assessing Preparedness Across Policy Dimensions

We start by considering the overlap between AVR and remote voting methods.[1] Table 5.1 shows the overlap between these two dimensions.

The most-common pairs on these two dimensions are excuse-required absentee voting and no-excuse absentee voting without AVR. States that offer no-excuse absentee voting, no-excuse absentee and

[1] Because North Dakota does not have voter registration, we include it as a "no AVR" state, but we note that voters are largely registered automatically on the basis of living in North Dakota.

Table 5.1
Remote Voting and AVR

Type of Remote Voting	No AVR	AVR
Excuse-required absentee	15	1
No-excuse absentee	15	6
No-excuse absentee and permanent mail-in	3	5
Universal mail-in (only)	2	3
Excuse-required absentee and no-excuse mail-in	1	0

SOURCE: National Conference of State Legislatures, 2020c; National Conference of State Legislatures, 2020d.

permanent mail-in, or universal mail-in are more likely to have AVR than states that offer excuse-required absentee voting.

We can better assess which states are more or less flexible across these two dimensions by considering all states with a no-excuse mail-in option together. States that offer no-excuse absentee, permanent mail-in, or universal mail-in options are more similar than different in their approach to remote voting. Essentially, these states offer a remote option for all eligible voters, although they differ on the actions that voters must take to get access to the absentee ballot. Table 5.2 groups these states into four categories, with the majority falling into one of three. About one-third of states (about 46 million registered voters) have no AVR and have excuse-required absentee voting. States adhering to these policies have the least flexibility to shift to remote and distributed processes and thus might be the least prepared for the requirements of voting during a pandemic. Almost one-third of states (about 49 million registered voters) allows for a no-excuse mail-in option of some kind and AVR. These states might already have much of the infrastructure that they need to support an increase in remote voting and already have the ability to register people using existing records. Finally, just under one-half of states (about 54.5 million registered voters) offer a no-excuse mail-in option without AVR.[2] These states

[2] Data on population by state were taken from World Population Review, undated.

Table 5.2
Remote Voting and AVR, Consolidated

Type of Remote Voting	No AVR	AVR
Mail-in option, no-excuse absentee	21	14[a]
Excuse-required absentee	15	1

SOURCE: National Conference of State Legislatures, 2020c; National Conference of State Legislatures, 2020d.

[a] The District of Columbia is included in this number.

fall somewhere in between the first two groups in terms of flexibility on the registration and remote voting dimensions. Only one state (Massachusetts) offers AVR and only excuse-required absentee voting, (in 2020, however, no-excuse mail-in voting will be available in Massachusetts).[3] West Virginia will also be in this group once its AVR legislation is implemented in 2021. Figure 5.1 shows the geographic distribution of these five categories.

There are a few interesting patterns in the relationship between remote and early voting methods (Table 5.3). First, almost all states that have some mail-in option also have early voting. Table 5.4 illustrates that more than 60 percent of states (about 97 million registered voters) offer some sort of mail-in option and early voting.[4] On these two dimensions, then, these states have the most flexibility—they can spread in-person voting attendance over multiple days, and they have an easy way to ensure that voters can submit ballots remotely. Only Pennsylvania and Rhode Island have no early voting but do have a no-excuse mail-in option. For states that have only excuse-required absentee voting, most offer some form of early voting, though six states offer early voting only to those with excuses. Three states have excuse-required absentee voting and no early voting: Alabama, Connecticut, and New Hampshire. Figure 5.2 shows the distribution of states using these consolidated characteristics.

[3] State of Massachusetts, H. 4820, Ch. 115 of the Acts of 2020, An Act Relative to Voting Options in Response to COVID-19, July 2, 2020.

[4] Data on population by state were taken from World Population Review, undated.

Figure 5.1
States by Remote Voting and AVR

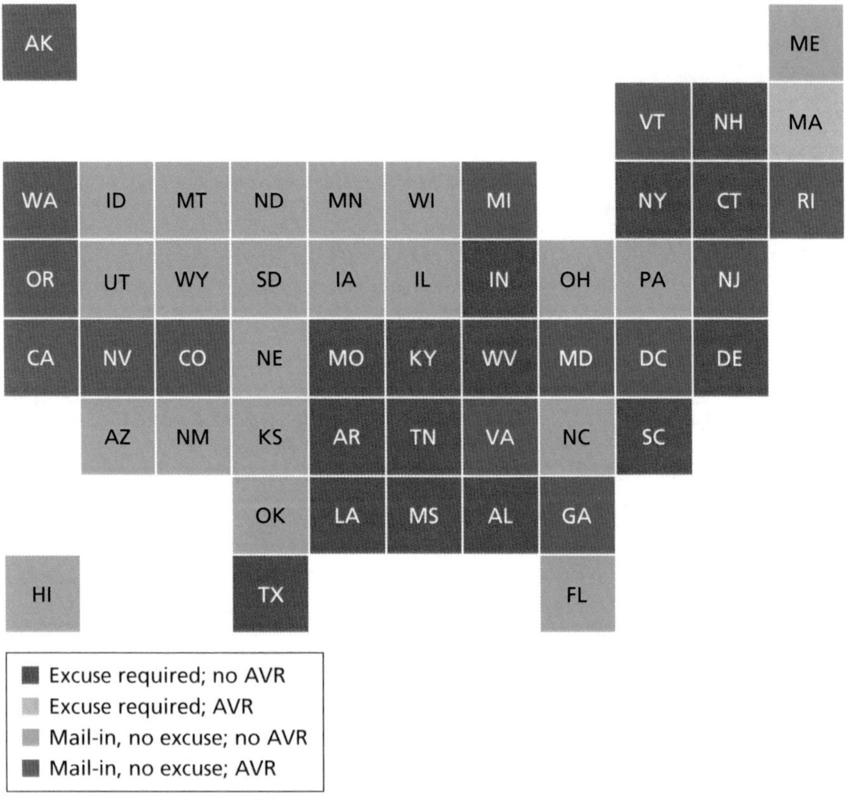

SOURCE: National Conference of State Legislatures, 2020c; National Conference of State Legislatures, 2020d.
NOTE: Because North Dakota does not have voter registration, we include it here as a "no AVR" state, but we note that voters are largely registered automatically on the basis of living in North Dakota. Pennsylvania also has an excuse-required absentee option.

Table 5.3
Remote Voting and Early Voting

Type of Remote Voting	Early Voting	No Early Voting	Excuse-Required
Excuse-required absentee	7	3	6
Excuse-required absentee and no-excuse mail-in	0	1	0
No-excuse absentee	20[a]	1	0
No-excuse absentee and permanent mail-in	8	0	0
Universal mail-in (only)	5	0	0

SOURCE: National Conference of State Legislatures, 2019b; National Conference of State Legislatures, 2020d.

[a] The District of Columbia is included in this number.

Table 5.4
Remote Voting and Early Voting, Consolidated

Type of Remote Voting	Early Voting	No Early Voting	Excuse-Required
Excuse-required absentee	7	3	6
Mail-in option	33[a]	2	0

SOURCE: National Conference of State Legislatures, 2019b; National Conference of State Legislatures, 2020d.

[a] The District of Columbia is included in this number.

Figure 5.2
States by Remote Voting and Early Voting

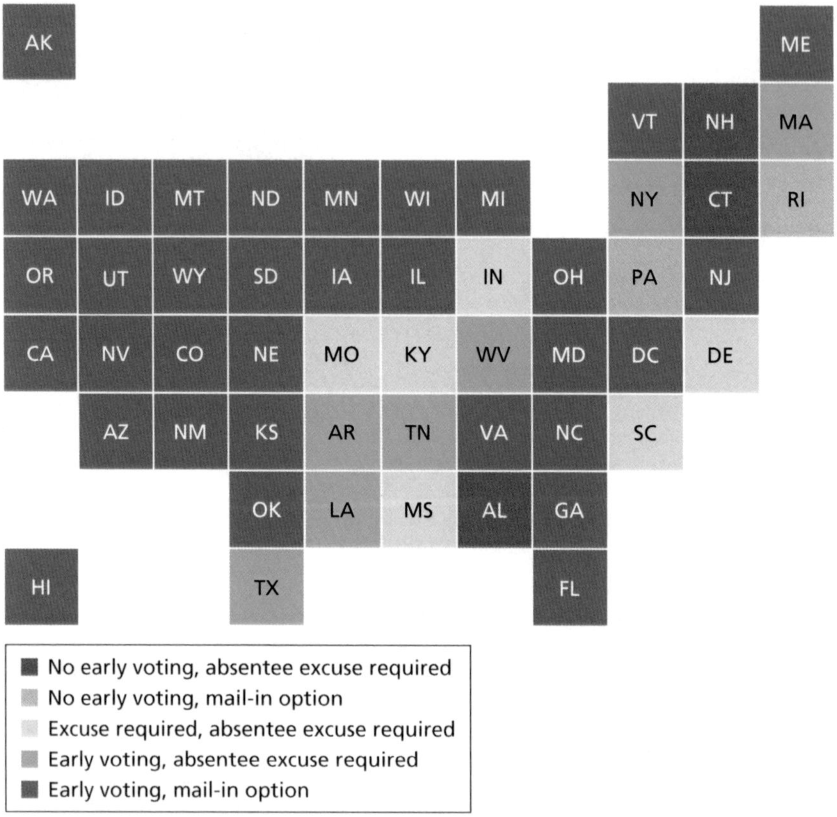

SOURCE: National Conference of State Legislatures, 2019b; National Conference of State Legislatures, 2020d.

Figure 5.3 and Table 5.5 illustrate the overlap across all three polices considered in this report. For simplicity, we collapse all the states with no-excuse mail-in options for this analysis. A few points are worth noting:

- All states with excuse-only early voting and most states with no early voting also have excuse-required absentee voting and no AVR. These nine states (accounting for about 18 million registered voters) favor in-person voting on Election Day and require

Figure 5.3
States by AVR, Remote Voting, and Early Voting

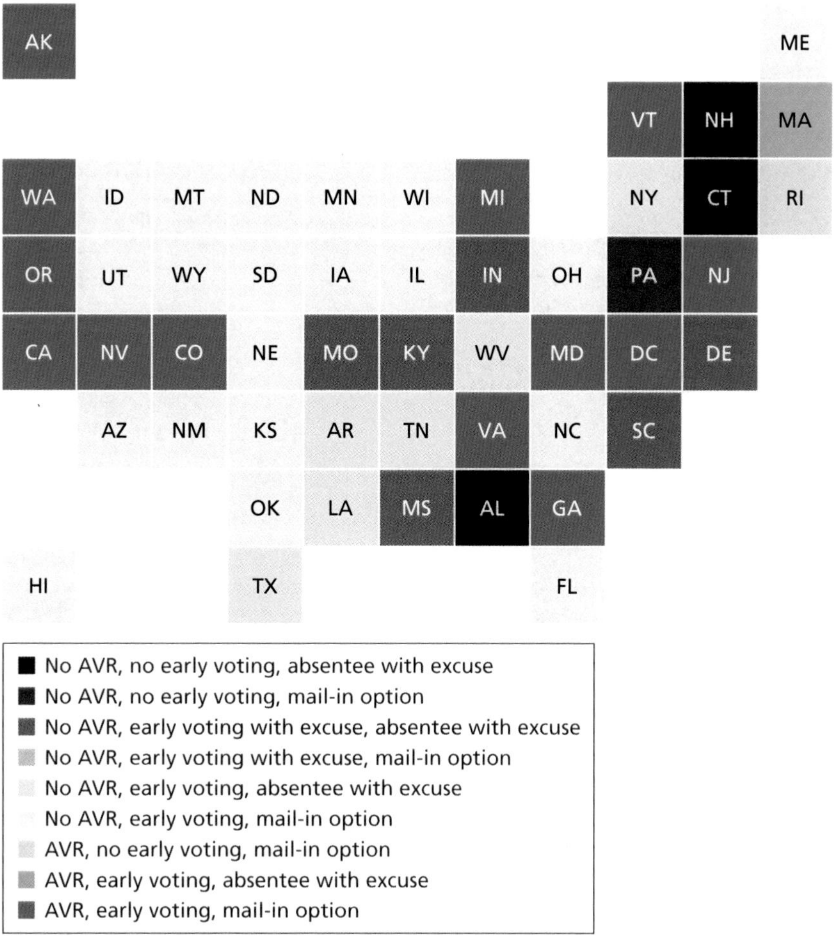

SOURCE: National Conference of State Legislatures, 2019b; National Conference of State Legislatures, 2020c; National Conference of State Legislatures, 2020d.
NOTE: Because North Dakota does not have voter registration, we include it here as a "no AVR" state, but we note that voters are largely registered automatically on the basis of living in North Dakota.

Table 5.5
AVR, Remote Voting, and Early Voting, Consolidated

	AVR			No AVR		
Type of Remote Voting	Early Voting	No Early Voting	Excuse-Required	Early Voting	No Early Voting	Excuse-Required
Excuse-required absentee	1	0	0	6	3	6
No-excuse mail-in option	13[a]	1	0	20	1	0

SOURCE: National Conference of State Legislatures, 2019b; National Conference of State Legislatures, 2020c; National Conference of State Legislatures, 2020d.

NOTE: Because North Dakota does not have voter registration, we include it here as a "no AVR" state, but we note that voters are largely registered automatically on the basis of living in North Dakota.

[a] The District of Columbia is included in this number.

that voters take additional active steps to register. They have the least flexibility for shifting voting processes to accommodate the requirements of the pandemic and will likely face a more significant challenge under COVID-19 conditions.

- More than one-third of states (about 49 million voters) with a no-excuse mail-in option also have early voting and AVR. These 12 states and the District of Columbia might be among those best postured for conducting an election under pandemic conditions because they already have a remote voting option, early voting to spread Election Day crowds, and AVR.
- Six states have excuse-required absentee voting and early voting but lack AVR.

Comparing Levels of Flexibility

In our analysis, we focused on specific policies used by different states to provide insight into how much flexibility individual states have on the three dimensions of the voting process considered in this report.[5] We can also use the summary assessments of flexibility presented in previous

5 As a reminder, unlike in the analysis focused on specific policies, here we include states that have opt-in, point-of-transaction registration options (such as Connecticut and Utah)

chapters to provide a more holistic assessment of flexibility that extends across dimensions. The advantage of this approach is that it incorporates additional pieces of the election process that can contribute to a state's ability to conduct elections during a pandemic by reducing person-to-person contact or facilitating remote processes beyond the three policies. As a reminder, we categorized states into one of four groups based on the flexibility of their voter registration, remote voting, and early voting processes: high, moderate, low, and none. For the sake of simplicity, in this analysis, we combine states that have no flexibility with those that have low flexibility and states that have high flexibility with those that have moderate flexibility. Table 5.6 shows how states fall across these three dimensions. There are a few relevant observations:

- Nine states (about 45 million registered voters) appear at the high end on all three dimensions and have the most flexibility on these three policies; these states are perhaps the best situated to deal with the challenges of conducting elections during a pandemic.

Table 5.6
Flexibility for Pandemic Preparedness Across Dimensions

Voter Registration	Remote Voting	Early Voting	Summary	Number of States
H	H	H	High	9
L	H	H	Moderate	10
H	H	L		10[a]
H	L	H		2
L	H	L	Low	4
L	L	H		0
H	L	L		4
L	L	L	Very Low	12

[a] The District of Columbia is included in this number.

and North Dakota alongside AVR as having the same pandemic-related flexibility (in reducing in-person transactions).

- Twelve states (about 30 million registered voters) at the very lowest end have the least flexibility to shift to remote processes and to reduce person-to-person contact. With one exception, these states have little flexibility in their voter registration process, excuse-required remote voting, and no early voting.
- Twenty-one states (about 43 million registered voters) and the District of Columbia have a high degree of flexibility across two of the three dimensions. For the most part, these states have easily accessible remote voting options, but about half have limited flexibility in voter registration; the other half lack early voting or have early voting that is open for less than two weeks.
- Eight states have high flexibility on only one dimension. Perhaps most interesting are those states with flexibility only in their registration process. They likely can navigate the challenges of registering voters remotely but might have less capacity to address challenges to the balloting process under COVID-19 restrictions. There are no states with highly flexible early voting options that do not also offer either flexible voter registration processes or easily accessible remote voting.
- Only one state, Mississippi, fell into the "no flexibility" category across dimensions.

Table 5.6 and Figure 5.4 display states along this aggregated metric of flexibility.

It is useful to consider the mix of states that fall in each of these four categories. Table 5.7 lists the states in each category. Again, we grouped states using a summary measure of state election policies' flexibility specifically in terms of shifting to remote processes and supporting social distancing. It is worth noting that both the most- and least-flexible groups of states are diverse in terms of size and geographic location. Several states favoring in-person processes and voting on Election Day are in the South, but some are in the Northeast, such as Delaware and New Hampshire. There are, however, few states in the Western half of the country on this list. States with more flexibility for remote processes and early voting are in the West, Midwest, and Northeast. The same is true of both the moderate and low groups.

Figure 5.4
Flexibility for Pandemic Preparedness Across Dimensions

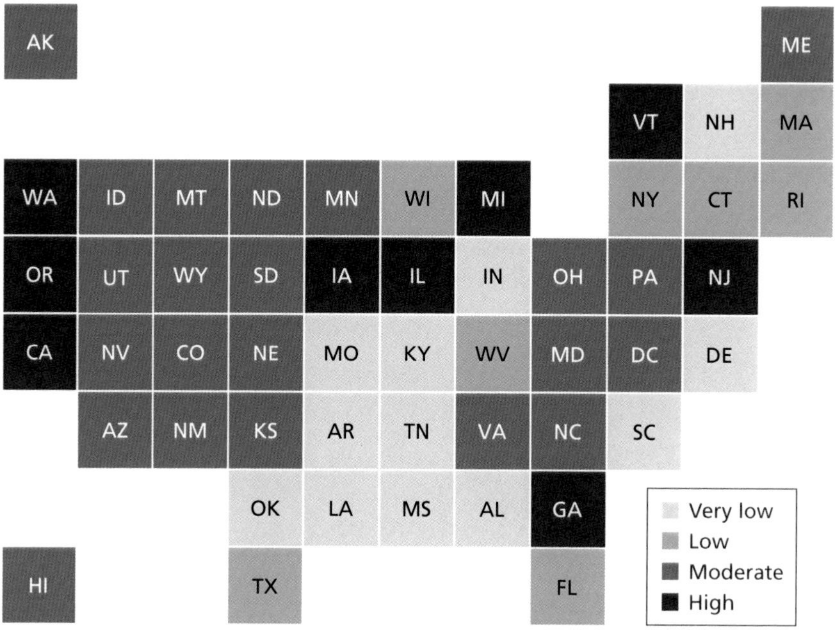

Table 5.7 can be useful in identifying which states are already well positioned for a shift to remote voting during a pandemic and which could have large challenges or require additional resources to make this transition. However, even the states in the "high flexibility" group might not have all the measures identified in this report as supporting preparedness. Only one state, Illinois, qualifies as highly flexible on all three dimensions (registration, remote voting, and early voting). Almost every state has options to pursue to make election processes more robust to potential COVID-19–related shocks in November. For some states, the short amount of time until the November election places some of these options out of reach, but this analysis can help states identify what options they do have.

This analysis has focused on the permanent voting procedures in place in the 50 states and the District of Columbia. However, a number of states have already instituted temporary provisions for the November 2020 general election as a result of the ongoing COVID-19 pan-

Table 5.7
States by Flexibility for Pandemic Preparedness

High	Moderate	Low	Very Low
California	Alaska	Connecticut	Alabama
Georgia	Arizona	Florida	Arkansas
Illinois	Colorado	Massachusetts	Delaware
Iowa	District of Columbia	New York	Indiana
Michigan	Idaho	Rhode Island	Kentucky
New Jersey	Hawaii	Texas	Louisiana
Oregon	Kansas	West Virginia	Mississippi
Vermont	Maine	Wisconsin	Missouri
Washington	Maryland		New Hampshire
	Minnesota		Oklahoma
	Montana		South Carolina
	Nebraska		Tennessee
	Nevada		
	New Mexico		
	North Carolina		
	North Dakota		
	Ohio		
	Pennsylvania		
	South Dakota		
	Utah		
	Virginia		
	Wyoming		

demic. It is worth noting that although there are many things that election officials can do to better prepare for the challenges of executing an election during a pandemic, implementing such temporary provisions as these usually requires actions by the state legislature or executive. States vary in their abilities and willingness to adopt such temporary procedures, based on political, legal, and logistical concerns. These provisions will better position these states to carry out safe elections in a pandemic context in 2020 but will not provide longer-term resilience to future pandemics or similarly disruptive situations. Table 5.8 lists temporary provisions in place as of July 27, 2020.

Table 5.8
Temporary Changes to State Election Procedures for the 2020 General Election

State	Description of Change to November 2020 Election Procedure
Alabama	No changes
Alaska	No changes
Arizona	No changes
Arkansas	For November 2020, concerns about COVID-19 can be cited as a valid excuse for absentee voting.
California	Mail-in ballots will be sent to all registered voters for the November 3, 2020, general election.
Colorado	No changes
Connecticut	Mail-in ballot applications will be sent to all registered voters for the November 3, 2020, general election.
Delaware	Mail-in ballot applications will be sent to all registered voters for the November 3, 2020, general election.
District of Columbia	Mail-in ballots will be sent to all registered voters for the November 3, 2020, general election. Additional early vote locations will be added.
Florida	No changes
Georgia	No changes
Hawaii	No changes
Idaho	Implementation of online process for requesting mail-in ballots.
Illinois	Mail-in ballot applications will be sent to all registered voters for the November 3, 2020, general election.
Indiana	No changes
Iowa	No changes
Kansas	No changes
Kentucky	No changes
Louisiana	No changes
Maine	No changes
Maryland	Mail-in ballot applications sent automatically to all voters for the November 3, 2020, general election.
Massachusetts	Absentee/mail-in voting eligibility extended to all qualified voters for the November 3, 2020, general election.
Michigan	Mail-in ballot applications sent automatically to all voters for the November 3, 2020, general election.
Minnesota	No changes
Mississippi	No changes

Table 5.8—Continued

State	Description of Change to November 2020 Election Procedure
Missouri	Absentee/mail-in voting eligibility extended to all qualified voters for the November 3, 2020, general election with requirement that completed ballot is notarized. Those who have contracted COVID-19 or are at higher risk for contracting the virus, are exempted from the notarization requirement.
Montana	No changes
Nebraska	No changes
Nevada	No changes
New Hampshire	Absentee/mail-in voting eligibility in the November 3, 2020, general election extended to any registered voter unable to vote in person because they are sick with COVID-19 or fear that voting in person may result in COVID-19 exposure for self or others.
New Jersey	No changes
New Mexico	Mail-in ballot applications sent automatically to all voters for the November 3, 2020, general election.
New York	No changes
North Carolina	Witness signature requirement for completed absentee ballots reduced from two to one for the November 3, 2020, general election.
North Dakota	No changes
Ohio	No changes
Oklahoma	Individuals experiencing symptoms of COVID-19 and individuals classified as "high risk" of infection can apply for absentee ballots under "physical incapacitation" eligibility criterion. Voters can submit copies of their identification in lieu of fulfilling the absentee ballot notarization requirement.
Oregon	No changes
Pennsylvania	No changes
Rhode Island	No changes
South Carolina	No changes
South Dakota	No changes
Tennessee	Absentee/mail-in voting eligibility extended to all qualified voters for the November 3, 2020, general election.
Texas	Early vote period extended by one week.
Utah	No changes
Vermont	No changes
Virginia	No changes
Washington	No changes
West Virginia	No changes
Wisconsin	No changes
Wyoming	No changes

SOURCE: Ballotpedia, "Changes to Election Dates, Procedures, and Administration in Response to the Coronavirus (COVID-19) Pandemic, 2020," webpage, undated.

CHAPTER SIX

Concluding Thoughts

In this report, we underscore the diversity across states in terms of both how elections are conducted and the flexibility that states have built into these systems on issues of voter registration, remote voting and early voting. We considered a specific type of flexibility—that which can ease a shift to socially distanced in-person and remote registration and voting—because this flexibility can lend itself to preparedness for conducting elections under pandemic conditions. Although some states have this flexibility across all the dimensions considered here, others have flexibility on only one or two dimensions. Even within a given dimension, different states pursue flexibility in different ways using different policies and provisions. Although we were able to identify common types of states, every state has its own exceptions, processes, and procedures. North Dakota, for example, is unique in its lack of a voter registration system. Pennsylvania has both an excuse-required absentee option and a no-excuse mail-in option. Considering the geography of the policies examined reveals some interesting patterns as well. The Western part of the United States has states with some of the more-flexible options in such areas as AVR, remote voting, and early voting (such as Washington and Oregon). States with less flexibility in remote and early voting appear to be largely in the South (Mississippi, Alabama, and Arkansas) and in the Northeast (New Hampshire and Delaware), although neither region is homogenous.

In summarizing the status of state election laws on these three dimensions, this report provides state policymakers with a benchmark of where they stand relative to other states and suggests models for remote and early voting access that could be emulated. States are not locked into their voting processes for November 2020. Many still have time to modify their systems, if desired, and shift to remote processes that reduce person-to-person contact. The summary provides a snapshot of how states vary in their flexibility regarding remote and distributed registration and voting options. To the extent that having more-flexible options can provide resiliency to a greater range of COVID-19 scenarios, state preparedness for pandemic-related challenges to the November 2020 election also varies.

References

Armitage, Susie, "Handwriting Disputes Cause Headaches for Some Absentee Voters," Propublica, November 5, 2018.

Ballotpedia, "Changes to Election Dates, Procedures, and Administration in Response to the Coronavirus (COVID-19) Pandemic, 2020," webpage, undated. As of July 20, 2020:
https://ballotpedia.org/Changes_to_election_dates,_procedures,_and_administration_in_response_to_the_coronavirus_(COVID-19)_pandemic,_2020

Brennan Center for Justice, "Voting Laws Roundup 2020," webpage, undated. As of February 4, 2020:
https://www.brennancenter.org/our-work/research-reports/voting-laws-roundup-2020

Brennan Center for Justice, "Policy Differences of Automatic Voter Registration," expert brief, January 17, 2020.

Brito, Christopher, "CDC Director Says Potentially Worse Second Wave of Coronavirus Could Come Along with Flu Season," CBS News, April 23, 2020. As of May 25, 2020:
https://www.cbsnews.com/news/coronavirus-second-wave-cdc-director-robert-redfield-warning-flu-season/

Commonwealth of Pennsylvania, "Voting in Pennsylvania," webpage, undated. As of May 31, 2020:
https://www.pa.gov/guides/voting-and-elections/

Constitution of the Commonwealth of Pennsylvania, Article VII, Paragraph 14, "Absentee Voting." As of June 1, 2020:
https://www.legis.state.pa.us/WU01/LI/LI/CT/HTM/00/00.HTM

Corse, Alexa, "Voting by Mail to Face Biggest Test Since Pandemic Started," *Wall Street Journal*, June 1, 2020.

Franklin, Daniel P., and Eric E. Grier, "Effects of Motor Voter Legislation: Voter Turnout, Registration, and Partisan Advantage in the 1992 Presidential Election," *American Politics Quarterly*, Vol. 25, No. 1, 1997, pp. 104–117.

Goel, Sharad, Marc Meredith, Michael Morse, David Rothschild, and Houshmand Shirani-Mehr, "One Person, One Vote: Estimating the Prevalence of Double Voting in U.S. Presidential Elections," *American Political Science Review*, Vol. 114, No. 2, May 2020, pp. 456–469.

"Governor Lamont Signs Executive Order Allowing All Eligible Connecticut Residents to Vote Absentee in August 11 Primary Elections," Office of Governor Ned Lamont, press release, May 20, 2020. As of June 20, 2020:
https://portal.ct.gov/Office-of-the-Governor/News/Press-Releases/2020/05-2020/Governor-Lamont-Signs-Executive-Order-Allowing-All-Eligible-Connecticut-Residents-to-Vote-Absentee

"Gov. Wolf Signs Executive Order Extending Mail Ballot Deadline in Six Counties to June 9," Governor Tom Wolf Newsroom, press release, June 1, 2020. As of June 20, 2020:
https://www.governor.pa.gov/newsroom/gov-wolf-signs-executive-order-extending-mail-ballot-deadline-in-six-counties-to-june-9/

Gronke, Paul, Eva Galanes-Rosenbaum, and Peter A. Miller, "Early Voting and Turnout," *PS: Political Science & Politics*, Vol. 40, No. 4, 2007, pp. 639–645.

Higgins, Tucker, "US Supreme Court Sides with GOP in Wisconsin: Absentee Ballots Must Be Sent by Tuesday," CNBC, April 6, 2020. As of June 20, 2020:
https://www.cnbc.com/2020/04/06/wisconsin-supreme-court-halts-absentee-ballot-deadline-extension.html

Hodgson, Quentin E., Jennifer Kavanagh, Anusree Garg, Edward W. Chan, and Christine Sovak, *Options for Ensuring Safe Elections: Preparing for Elections During a Pandemic*, Santa Monica, Calif.: RAND Corporation, RR-A112-10, 2020. As of August 2020:
https://www.rand.org/pubs/research_reports/RRA112-10.html

Itkowitz, Colby, and Amy Gardner, "New Hampshire Governor to Allow Absentee Voting in November Because of Coronavirus Outbreak," *Washington Post*, April 9, 2020.

Kamarck, Elaine, and Christine Stenglein, "Low Rates of Fraud in Vote-by-Mail States Show the Benefits Outweigh the Risks," Brookings Institution, June 2, 2020. As of June 20, 2020:
https://www.brookings.edu/blog/fixgov/2020/06/02/low-rates-of-fraud-in-vote-by-mail-states-show-the-benefits-outweigh-the-risks/

Karp, Jeffrey A., and Susan A. Banducci, "Going Postal: How All-Mail Elections Influence Turnout," *Political Behavior*, Vol. 22, No. 3, 2000, pp. 223–239.

Kavanagh, Jennifer, C. Ben Gibson, and Samantha Cherney, *Database of State Voting Laws: Preparing for Elections During a Pandemic,* Santa Monica, Calif.: RAND Corporation, TL-A112-1, 2020. As of August 2020:
https://www.rand.org/pubs/tools/TLA112-1.html

Kavanagh, Jennifer, and Michael D. Rich, *Truth Decay: An Initial Exploration of the Diminishing Role of Facts and Analysis in American Public Life*, Santa Monica, Calif., RAND Corporation, RR-2314-RC: 2018. As of July 14, 2020: https://www.rand.org/pubs/research_reports/RR2314.html

Kissler, Stephen M., Christine Tedijanto, Edward Goldstein, Yonatan H. Grad, and Marc Lipsitch, "Projecting the Transmission Dynamics of SARS-CoV-2 Through the Postpandemic Period," *Science*, Vol. 368, No. 6493, 2020, pp. 860–868. As of June 19, 2020: https://science.sciencemag.org/content/368/6493/860

Minnite, Lori, and David Callahan, *Securing the Vote*, New York: Demos, 2003.

Moore, Kristine A., Marc Lipsitch, John M. Barry, and Michael T. Osterholm, *COVID-19: The CIDRAP Viewpoint*, Part 1, *The Future of the COVID-19 Pandemic: Lessons Learned from Pandemic Influenza*, Minneapolis, Minn.: Center for Infectious Disease Research and Policy, University of Minnesota, April 30, 2020. As of May 25, 2020: https://www.cidrap.umn.edu/sites/default/files/public/downloads/cidrap-covid19-viewpoint-part1_0.pdf

National Academies of Sciences, Engineering, and Medicine, *Securing the Vote: Protecting American Democracy*, Washington, D.C.: National Academies Press, 2018.

National Conference of State Legislatures, "Same Day Voter Registration," webpage, June 28, 2019a. As of June 20, 2020: https://www.ncsl.org/research/elections-and-campaigns/same-day-registration.aspx

National Conference of State Legislatures, "State Laws Governing Early Voting," webpage, August 2, 2019b. As of June 20, 2020: https://www.ncsl.org/research/elections-and-campaigns/early-voting-in-state-elections.aspx

National Conference of State Legislatures, "Verification of Absentee Ballots," webpage, January 21, 2020a. As of June 20, 2020: https://www.ncsl.org/research/elections-and-campaigns/verification-of-absentee-ballots.aspx

National Conference of State Legislatures, "Online Voter Registration," webpage, February 3, 2020b. As of June 20, 2020: https://www.ncsl.org/research/elections-and-campaigns/electronic-or-online-voter-registration.aspx

National Conference of State Legislatures, "Automatic Voter Registration," webpage, April 14, 2020c. As of June 20, 2020: https://www.ncsl.org/research/elections-and-campaigns/automatic-voter-registration.aspx

National Conference of State Legislatures, "Voting Outside the Polling Place: Absentee, All-Mail and Other Voting at Home Options," webpage, June 9, 2020d. As of June 20, 2020:
https://www.ncsl.org/research/elections-and-campaigns/absentee-and-early-voting.aspx

National Conference of State Legislatures, "Receipt and Postmark Deadlines for Absentee Ballots," webpage, June 15, 2020e. As of June 20, 2020:
https://www.ncsl.org/research/elections-and-campaigns/vopp-table-11-receipt-and-postmark-deadlines-for-absentee-ballots.aspx

New Jersey Executive Order 105, March 9, 2020. As of June 23, 2020:
https://nj.gov/infobank/eo/056murphy/pdf/EO-105.pdf

Norden, Lawrence, Edgardo Cortés, Elizabeth Howard, Derek Tisler, and Gowri Ramachandran, *Estimated Costs of COVID-19 Election Resiliency Measures*, New York: Brennan Center for Justice, April 18, 2020. As of June 20, 2020:
https://www.brennancenter.org/our-work/research-reports/estimated-costs-covid-19-election-resiliency-measures

Phillips, Amber, "Examining the Arguments Against Voting by Mail," *Washington Post*, May 20, 2020.

"Rush to Vote-by-Mail Requires Decisions on Signature Verification," Global Newswire, April 23, 2020.

Secretary of State North Dakota, "ID Required for Voting," webpage, undated-a. As of May 31, 2020:
https://vip.sos.nd.gov/IDRequirements.aspx?ptlhPKID=103&ptlPKID=7

Secretary of State North Dakota, "When Do Eligible Voters Register for an Election?" webpage, undated-b. As of June 15, 2020:
https://vip.sos.nd.gov/PortalListDetails.aspx?ptlhPKID=79&ptlPKID=7

Southwell, Priscilla L., and Justin I. Burchett, "The Effect of All-Mail Elections on Voter Turnout," *American Politics Quarterly*, Vol. 28, No. 1, 2000, pp. 72–79.

State of Massachusetts, H. 4820, Ch. 115 of the Acts of 2020, An Act Relative to Voting Options in Response to COVID-19, July 2, 2020. As of July 13, 2020:
http://cdn.cnn.com/cnn/2020/images/07/07/h4820.signed.pdf

State of Rhode Island Board of Elections, "Mail Ballot," webpage, undated. As of June 2, 2020:
https://elections.ri.gov/voting/mailballot.php

Stein, Robert M., "Introduction: Early Voting," *Public Opinion Quarterly*, Vol. 62, No. 1, 1998, pp. 57–69.

Stein, Robert M., *The Incidence and Detection of Ineligible Voting*, paper presented at the American Political Science Association 2013 annual meeting, 2013.

U.S. Department of Justice, "The Uniformed and Overseas Citizens Absentee Voting Act," webpage, February 26, 2020. As of June 20, 2020:
https://www.justice.gov/servicemembers/uniformed-and-overseas-citizens-absentee-voting-act-uocava

Vote Riders, "Voter ID for Absentee Ballots," webpage, undated. As of May 31, 2020:
https://www.voteriders.org/voter-id-for-absentee-ballots/

Wines, Michael, "Covid-19 Changed How We Vote. It Could Also Change Who Votes," *New York Times*, June 14, 2020. As of June 15, 2020:
https://www.nytimes.com/2020/06/14/us/voter-registration-coronavirus-2020-election.html

World Population Review, "Number of Registered Voters by State 2020," webpage, undated. As of June 10, 2020:
https://worldpopulationreview.com/states/number-of-registered-voters-by-state/

About the Authors

Jennifer Kavanagh is a senior political scientist at the RAND Corporation and director of the Strategy, Doctrine, and Resources Program in the RAND Arroyo Center. She also leads RAND's Countering Truth Decay initiative, a portfolio of projects exploring the diminishing reliance on facts and analysis in U.S. political and civil discourse. Her research focuses on U.S. defense strategy, international conflict, disinformation, and the relationship between U.S. political and media institutions. She earned her Ph.D. in political science and public policy.

Quentin E. Hodgson is a senior international and defense researcher at the RAND Corporation focusing on cybersecurity, cyber operations, critical infrastructure protection, risk management, and command and control. He has led projects for the Department of Defense, the Department of Homeland Security, and NATO's Allied Command Transformation. He holds an M.A. in international relations and an M.Sc. in national resource management, and was a Fulbright scholar affiliated with the University of Potsdam, Germany.

C. Ben Gibson is an associate behavioral/social scientist at the RAND Corporation. He has interests in conversation analysis, rumoring, information diffusion, and consensus formation; diffusion modeling in social networks; cybersecurity (both human factors and threat detection); statistical methodology, especially computational modeling of networks and other relational dynamics; informant accuracy and survey methods; and international conflict. He holds a Ph.D. in sociology.

Samantha Cherney is a quantitative analyst at the RAND Corporation. Her research portfolio includes work on civil and criminal justice, insurance, and army contracting and on RAND's Gun Policy in America initiative. Cherney received a J.D. in 2011, and she is a licensed attorney in New York and New Jersey.